MENTAL HEALTH
THE ROLE OF THE APPROVED SOCIAL WORKER

MICHAEL SHEPPARD

CONTENTS

Preface v

PART ONE: APPROVED SOCIAL WORKERS AS GATEKEEPERS 1

PART TWO: ASSESSMENT FOR COMPULSORY ADMISSIONS BY ASWs 36

PART THREE: A SCHEDULE FOR ASSESSING COMPULSORY ADMISSIONS 76

PART FOUR: THE ROLE OF THE ASW IN CONTEXT 118

References 156

PREFACE

This book attempts to increase social work knowledge in one particular, but crucial, area of practice: that relating to the assessment of individuals for possible compulsory admission to mental hospitals under the Mental Health Act. It is an area of special interest for social work. When making such assessments practitioners are involved in weighty issues relating to freedom and confinement, and when they do so they act as independent professionals rather than agency representatives. It can be a very complex and difficult exercise, one which merits advanced training required to achieve competence in approved social work.

Although hinging on research undertaken on the work of approved social workers, it aims to produce something of use to practice. In this respect the book's most important innovation is the Compulsory Admission Assessment Schedule, which the reader will find at the end of Part Three. A description of the Schedule and instructions on how to use it form the bulk of Part Three. It is the author's hope that it will be adopted by approved social workers for use in their assessments. It is particularly aimed, in addition, at approved social worker training courses. Aspiring ASWs can both analyse cases and learn how to use the schedule while undergoing their training, perhaps by the use of case examples or vignettes, or when accompanying ASWs when undertaking section assessments.

In addition to developing the knowledge base of social work, the book aims to clarify the role of the ASW. This is an important issue, for the ASW may be perceived as the 'poor man's (or woman's) psychiatrist' or simply as an adjunct to the medical practitioners involved. This is most emphatically not the case as will, I hope, become apparent in the course of the book. ASWs have a distinctive and important role to play when making compulsory admission assessments, one which calls upon the use of knowledge and skills which are, taken together, recognisably and distinctively those of social work.

The book is divided into four parts. The first part draws together some aspects of what we already know about compulsory admissions, and develops the notion of the ASW as gatekeeper. This provides the groundwork for demonstrating the importance, in a societal context, of the ASW role. It also examines some key concepts of risk analysis which will be used throughout the rest of the book. Part Two uses risk analysis to examine in detail the practice of ASWs in relation to compulsory admission assessments. It is argued that the criteria of 'health or safety of the patient' or 'protection of other persons' provide the key to understanding the ASW role. Social work practice is shown in some respects to be problematic, and the key to developing good practice, it is argued, is the development amongst ASWs of a 'social risk' orientation. Part Three develops the major elements of the Compulsory Admissions Assessment Schedule, which may be used to assess the criteria of health or safety of the patient or protection of other persons, and which represents the practical application of a 'social risk' orientation. Finally, Part Four examines a number of outstanding issues about the role of ASWs, their relationship with medical practitioners, the importance of the concept of social functioning, and the (anomalous) position of the nearest relative.

This book also attempts to break new ground in the approach it takes to knowledge development. A great deal of excellent work has been produced, based on research projects, which provides useful guidelines to practitioners. This book, however, attempts to go one stage further by creating a direct relationship between the empirical research and conceptual developments and practice through the Compulsory Admission Assessment Schedule. The Schedule is, to a considerable degree, the actual embodiment of the concepts and research developed in this book. The principles on which this transmission from 'theory' to 'practice' is undertaken are discussed at the beginning of Part Three and in a section of Part Four. I believe that assessment schedules - not to be confused with mere checklists - could provide one useful way forward for social work, particularly in carrying out assessments.

The research which forms a core element of this book was not a matter of a researcher swooping down from cloistered academia to subject a group of ASWs to close examination. It was a joint project, and if it contains any merit, much of the credit is theirs. It takes an extremely brave practitioner to allow their practice to be subject to such close analysis. It also involves a commitment to high professional standards, through a preparedness to examine and improve their practice. As an ASW myself, I am aware at first hand of the enormous difficulties and dilemmas that are confronted in practice. I would like, therefore, to thank those involved for their participation. I hope the outcome justifies their commitment. Enterprises such as this one are always collaborative.

I would like also to thank my wife Margaret for her support while I wrote this. Anyone who wishes to know its contents should ask her. She was subject, as usual, to the development of my ideas above and beyond the call of duty. My two typists, Barbara Ham and Dorothy Templeman, showed great patience as I asked them to type and retype the text.

Finally, I would like to thank Martin Davies and David Howe for their support when I was trying to get into a position where I could undertake this kind of research. I hope this provides at least partial repayment for their confidence.

PART ONE

APPROVED SOCIAL WORKERS AS GATEKEEPERS

Introduction

Social work in the mental health field has, as Fisher et al (1984) pointed out, received little attention in terms of research, a situation which contrasts sharply with the noticeable number of 'practice handbooks' which have been produced (Hudson, 1982; Butler and Pritchard, 1983; Munro and McCulloch, 1969). Much of the research has been in isolated articles (Hudson, 1974; Hudson, 1978; Huxley and Fitzpatrick, 1983), and although some useful material has appeared since Fisher and his colleagues wrote, this area remains singularly underdeveloped (Corney, 1984; Huxley et al, 1987).

The social work role is very wide in the realm of mental health where responsibilities normally include areas of prevention, detection, rehabilitation and support. Social workers may work closely (with greater or lesser success) with primary health care professionals, and the psychiatric and nursing professions in carrying out their duties. Furthermore, such work is not only carried out by specialist psychiatric social workers, or simply in mental health settings, since mental health issues frequently permeate other areas of work, such as those defined by the agency as child care or elderly work (Fisher et al, 1984). Indeed, the extent of psychiatric disturbance in the community is often underestimated (Goldberg and Huxley, 1980; Brown and Harris, 1978) and mental health issues often go unrecognised by social workers in area teams (Huxley et al, 1987).

It is arguable, however, that the most critical aspect of mental health social work relates to compulsory admissions, through which individuals diagnosed as mentally disordered may, in particular circumstances, be admitted against their will to mental hospital. Social workers approved under the Mental Health Act 1983 frequently play a key role in the process of admission and thus hold a great deal of power. This work therefore involves not just good practice, but the civil liberties of the individuals involved: hence it is a matter not just of professional interest but socio-legal concern. Particular questions arise: are the circumstances of admission such as to inspire confidence that legal rules are being appropriately applied? Are the rules being applied impartially and consistently, or are similar situations being treated differently? These produce secondary questions relating to the evaluation of practice: how able are Approved Social Workers (ASWs) to make competent judgements when assessing for compulsory admission? With what degree of clarity are assessments made? If there are weaknesses, how far is this the fault of the law? How far is it the result of the behaviour and assumptions of the professionals involved? And finally, are there ways in which practice may be improved? These are questions which will be addressed here.

The book will broadly be divided into four parts. First, we shall try to understand the function of social workers as ASWs, by conceptualising their role as that of gatekeeper, and examining how risk analysis, plus other theoretical considerations, provide a basis for analysing that role. Second, the behaviour of ASWs in relation to 120 assessments for compulsory admission will be analysed using risk analysis. Third, again within the framework of risk analysis, a framework will be developed for the assessment of individuals for possible compulsory admission. Finally, some comments will be made drawing these elements together. Throughout all this the focus will be on one of the two major sets of criteria when considering compulsory admission: 'The Health or Safety of the Patient' and the 'Protection of Other Persons', which, it will be argued, provides the key to the ASW role. It is undertaken on the basis that there is a close relationship between social work practice, the development of expertise, and the civil rights of the patients concerned.

The ASW and Compulsory Admissions

The Mental Health Act 1983 (the Act), like its predecessor the 1959 Act, involves major issues of civil rights insofar as it gives specific professionals - doctors, police and approved social workers (ASWs) - the right to admit individuals in particular circumstances and against their will to psychiatric hospitals. In fact the issues are endowed with even greater complexity because of the uneasy relationship between the perceived treatment needs of the patient, and his 'normal' rights to choose whether or not to obtain treatment.

In relation to compulsory admissions (sections), the Act confronts this in three ways: by providing criteria under which a person may be compulsorily admitted, by giving patients the right - except under Section

4 - to appeal, and by giving the nearest relative the right of discharge and also of appealing to the Mental Health Review Tribunal.

The first of these is of greatest concern here. The overwhelming majority of compulsory admissions are undertaken under Sections 2, 3 or 4 of the Act (Mental Health Act Commission, 1985; 1987). Although for different purposes, the *grounds* for these sections have common characteristics. First, the patient must be suffering from a mental disorder (Section 3 requires a more precise indication of the *type* of mental disorder) warranting detention in hospital for Assessment (Sections 2 and 4) or Treatment (Section 3). Second, this should occur for the 'Health or Safety' of the patient or the 'Protection of Other Persons'. Third, there must be an application - by an ASW or nearest relative - accompanied by a medical recommendation by one (Section 4) or two (Sections 2 and 3) medical practitioners.

Thus the critical criteria in relation to sections are the presence or absence of mental disorder, and the health or safety of the patient and protection of others considerations. Both are poorly defined, with little direct guidance in the Act. While, however, mental disorder is left to clinical judgement, this may be justified in terms of the accumulated expertise and training of approved doctors. There is, however, little information about the circumstances under which we may state, for example, whether the health or safety of the patient is or is not at risk. The Act's rather bald statements on this issue leave it open to wide interpretation with, of course, major civil rights implications for the patient.

The ASW occupies a pivotal position in this process, as applicant in over 90% of admissions (Mental Health Act Commission, 1985). It is a highly significant area of social work practice, a point emphasised by the requirement of a minimum of two years post-qualified relevant experience, plus the completion of an advanced course before the worker may become an ASW. Indeed, the alarmed comments of examiners about some of the poorer examination performances further emphasises the concern for high quality practice (CCETSW, 1986).

The 1983 Act, furthermore, outlines rather better than its predecessor, the 1959 Act, a clear and important role for the ASW. This reflects to a considerable extent a recognition of the significance of social factors in mental illness, extensively chronicled in the social psychiatry literature (Cochrane, 1983) and the previously apparently limited analysis of social factors in assessment for compulsory admission (Bean, 1980). Thus, the ASW possesses a number of powers and duties, many of which reflect their position as 'social analysts', and inherent in powers such as those of entry and inspection (Section 115) and applying for a warrant to search for and remove patients (Section 135) where social factors (e.g. neglect, ill treatment, not being under proper care) are paramount. This is also evident from the DHSS memorandum (DHSS, 1983) which indicates social factors to be assessed to interview in a suitable manner (Section 13(2)). This involves considering 'all the circumstances' of the case: including, in addition to past and present state of mental disorder, the social, familial and personal factors relevant to the case. The ASW, therefore, has a distinctive role.

There are particular reasons why we should subject ASW practice in this area to detailed research. First, they have a special status under the Act; their authority arises from their status as ASWs rather than 'agency representatives', unique in local authority social work (see e.g. Section 13(3) and Section 139). Second, Bean (1980) suggests we should always be sceptical about groups who have power, especially when carried out without some external (e.g. court) oversight, and particularly where the exercise of this power involves the loss of liberty, and where those involved claim to operate in the subject's best interest.

Yet we have no idea how the central criteria of health or safety of the patient or protection of others is interpreted *in practice* by ASWs. Given the Act's loose formulation, this is a critical area of both social work and civil rights. It follows from this that detailed analysis of their interpretation and suggestions for the development of systematic, knowledge based assessment is of considerable importance. This is particularly the case in view of the, at times, crisis nature of the situations and the pressure that may be placed on ASWs by relatives, neighbours and doctors.

Indeed, in view of the importance of this area, it is surprising that more attention has not been given to the workings of the Act as a whole. At present published work is limited to a few brief articles (Edwards and Huxley, 1985; Bowl et al, 1987). There is considerably more work available on the 1959 Act, but it is unclear how much is now relevant, insofar as the 1983 Act was, in many respects, designed to curb the excesses of the 1959 Act, and specifically in relation to social work, additional training requirements have been established. Practice under the 1983 Act may vary greatly from that under the 1959 Act.

The research falls broadly into three categories. First, it examines the 'disposal' of patients assessed for compulsory admission, i.e. whether or not they were admitted, whether informally or compulsorily, and if compulsorily, under which section (Inechin et al, 1984; Smuckler et al, 1981; Edwards and Huxley, 1985). We are, however, fortunate here to have up to date figures superseding those previous studies focussing on the 1959 Act (Bowl et al, 1987). The data presented by Bowl, Barnes and Fisher show a slight reduction in compulsory admissions as a proportion of total admissions, and a rapid reduction in the proportion of total admissions undertaken as emergencies, following the 1983 Act (1982 - 47.8%; 1985-6 - 15.1%). While this may be welcomed, the lack of alternative resources meant those not sectioned were frequently admitted informally rather than directed to appropriate alternatives. Recent research suggests that this 'diversion' of patients away from compulsory admission was to a considerable degree the result of ASW intervention (Barnes et al, 1986; Fisher et al, 1987). This reflected a philosophy of adopting the 'least restrictive alternative'. Diversion effected out of hours showed more reliance on family and social work resources, while other formal medical and psychiatric resources were used during normal working hours.

Second, the research tries to identify which groups were most vulnerable to compulsory admission, by comparing them with informally admitted patients and placing them in the context of the general population. This has been undertaken both in terms of those *referred* for compulsory admission, and those *actually* compulsorily admitted. This has mainly focussed on urban areas and in relation to the 1959 Act (Smuckler et al, 1981; Harrison et al, 1984), although the most comprehensive and recent work has covered 42 urban and rural social service authorities in the use of the 1983 Act (Barnes et al, 1986; Fisher et al,1987; Bowl et al, 1987). In relation to gender, women are significantly more likely to be subject to assessment for compulsory admission, and when assessed are more likely to be admitted. The authors of one study (Barnes et al, in press) comment that:

> 'women may still find themselves subject to more subtle forms of control from the psychiatric profession that too often views mental distress in women as a result of their resistance to their familial role.'

A second key variable relates to race. Where ethnic factors are considered, Afro-Caribbeans, whether first or second generation, are considerably over represented, whether amongst offender or non-offender compulsory admissions (Sims and Symonds, 1975; Inechin et al, 1984; McGovern and Cope, 1987). Evidence to this effect has been demonstrated in relation to the 1959 Act in both London and Bristol (Smuckler et al, 1981; Inechin et al, 1984). More recent research on the 1983 Act demonstrates this to be the case over a wider area, including parts of London, the Midlands and West Yorkshire (Barnes et al, in press). Afro-Caribbeans were referred for compulsory admission nearly twice as frequently, relative to their population size, as the rate for the total population. Interestingly, the rate of referral for Asians was considerably lower than the rate for the whole population. Furthermore, once referred, Afro-Caribbeans were noticeably more likely than either white or Asian people to be compulsorily admitted. Great care should be taken when interpreting these figures. They do not necessarily indicate particular ethnic groups to be innately, or biologically, more subject to mental illness. Bowl, Barnes and Fisher (in press) suggest that:

> 'the cumulative effect of decisions made by these workers is indicative of a racist response to the mental health problems of those referred to them.'

However, this is not the only possibility. It may also indicate the effects of race hatred in the wider society, creating stress whose effects are to increase the incidence of mental illness amongst certain groups. Furthermore, Afro-Caribbeans as a whole are more deprived than the general population, suffering greater levels of unemployment, poor housing, poor education and generally living in poorer environments, all of which are associated with increased rates of mental illness (Sheppard, 1988).

Psychotic patients are considerably over-represented in compulsory admissions when compared with voluntary admissions and consistently, in the form generally of schizophrenia or affective psychosis, comprise a large majority of all compulsory admissions (Harrison et al, 1984; Fisher et al, 1984; Barnes et al, in press). Furthermore, in relation to urban areas the patients tend to come from deprived inner city districts and show a greater degree of social dislocation, are less settled and more transitory than informal admissions or the general population. Although this is particularly emphasised in relation to compulsory admission, this is a tendency also observed in ecological studies of psychotic patients in general who are more frequently found in the 'bedsit land' of inner cities which is characterised by a more drifting transitory population. This is the case also specifically in relation to police referrals for compulsory admissions (Sims and Symonds, 1975).

One factor linking these elements and which helps identify the 'at risk' population is patients' social isolation from the 'normal' active social life of the community. Women may be socially isolated by child care responsibilities and interaction limited to their partner; men have a tendency either not to have broken away from their family of birth or to have left their family but failed to forge new relationships. This social isolation is emphasised in one study by the huge number of patients unemployed: over half the women and nearly three quarters of the men aged under 55 were unemployed (Fisher et al, 1987).

Third, research has examined the process of admission (Clark, 1971; Smuckler, 1981; Bean, 1980; Fisher et al, 1984), or provided case descriptions (Christian, 1985). Certain common characteristics are evident. Sections are more likely with seriously disturbed patients, particularly where it involves social disturbance in a public place. These would be, for example, highly visible deviations from social norms, such as someone shouting threateningly at people in a busy thoroughfare, and slapping a complete stranger in the face (Smuckler, 1981; Bean, 1980). These may not be formally recognised by psychiatrists, but could be reinterpreted in terms of psychiatric symtomatology. Second, the patient is more likely to be sectioned rather than informally admitted where they actively or passively refuse to accept the patient role bestowed by the psychiatrist. Thus, where the choice was between informal and compulsory admission, informal admission occurred where both patient and doctor agreed the patient was ill and needed treatment, or when the patient at least acquiesced and accepted the patient role. Compulsory admission occurred when the psychiatrist ascribed to the person the patient role, and they either did not accept it or did not react at all. Third, some patients[*] in one study were sectioned according to their perceived needs regardless of legal rules: this somewhat cavalier attitude to the law meant in some circumstances that patients were admitted actually in contravention of the spirit, or worse, the letter of the law, where grounds did not exist for compulsory admission or the process of admission was illegal (Bean, 1980). Finally, discussions about admissions can involve some interprofessional tension. Under the 1959 Act, some psychiatrists accused social workers of being anti-psychiatric, disregarding the needs of patients, and of being incompetent. Social workers themselves admitted discomfort with mental illness, and some disquiet with their social control function in compulsory admission, but felt GPs frequently knew little of psychiatry *or* the law and often simply wished to 'dump' awkward patients on others (Fisher et al, 1984; Bean, 1980).

---

[*] The term 'patient' is used here in the same sense as defined in Section 145 of the Act. It is not used by the author as an insidious means of incorporating medical ideology into social work practice, but if we are to reflect the Act then this appears an appropriate term, despite its medical associations.

Smuckler (1981) concludes with a (value laden) typology of sectioned patients:

1. Chronic Psychotic Drifters
2. Chaotic Personality Disturbance
3. Marginally Socially Integrated
4. Socially Integrated

The ASW as Gatekeeper

In order to make sense, as Howe (1987) cogently argues, of what is going on in any social situation - and this applies to social work as much as other areas of social life - we need to have recourse to theory. Without it we are unguided: we do not know what we are looking at, how to look at it and where we are going in our analysis. It will become apparent, indeed, in the course of the book, how serious the lack of a theory-guided knowledge base may be for practice. The reader, however, may find this section a little tricky, although after this we shall enter the rather more familiar terrain of practice. It may, therefore, be helpful to provide a brief summary of the analysis before embarking on it in detail.

This section focusses on a description of the role of the ASW. The core of the analysis is that the ASW should be seen as a 'gatekeeper', because they are involved in a process where individuals (the patient) are given 'access' to particular identities (mental disorder) and resources (hospital). They possess this power, second, because it is delegated to them (as a profession) by the state through the Mental Health Act. The state is interested in this mental health issue, third, because it is a social problem; in certain circumstances the behaviour of some people considered mentally ill causes social concern. However, fourth, the law is not precise - a lack of precision which is called the 'open texture of law' - and because of this the ASW together with other involved professionals possesses a considerable degree of discretion to interpret individual circumstances and make decisions about whether or not someone should be compulsorily admitted to hospital. This gives ASWs a great deal of power.

This is the core of the analysis. The key elements of the ASW role are:

1. That unlike doctors, ASWs are concerned with mental health, under the Mental Health Act, as a *social* rather than health problem. This contrasts with the claims of medicine which are legitimated to a considerable degree by expertise in the arena of health.

2. ASWs act as gatekeeper in compulsory admission assessments.

3. They have a considerable degree of discretion in exercising their powers under the Act.

Before embarking on the analysis of the field data, it is necessary to obtain a clear idea of the nature and function of the ASW role. In so doing, it is possible to be clearer about the nature of the process undertaken and the importance attached to it. In asking the question 'What is the function of the ASW in their role as compulsory admission assessors?' a functionalist position is being adopted (Burrell and Morgan, 1979). This is because our concern is not with the validity of the ASW role itself, or with the state's power to define both the role and the problems which are its focus. In this respect, this corresponds closely with the situation, in practice, which confronts social workers. The very legitimacy of their action as ASWs depends upon the role conferred upon them by the state through specific legislation.

Indeed, this is a situation, it has been strongly argued, which characterises social work as a whole: that the profession is concerned with a disparate set of roles and responsibilities which arise only because of its position within social service agencies, the functions of those agencies, and laws which give social workers their responsibilities (Howe, 1980). Social workers are involved with matters of 'social concern' which are carried out under 'social auspices' (Howe, 1979); and they are, to a considerable extent, committed to consensus assumptions (Davies, 1985). If we are to provide research which is useful to ASWs we must reflect their concerns and interests.

The ASW may be usefully conceptualised as a 'gatekeeper': that is a person who is in a position to define the status of particular people (in terms of mental illness) and who can provide access to resources (hospital or other facilities). In so doing, they define some people 'into' a particular status and other people 'out'. They are not the only people in gatekeeping positions: doctors and the police are also. Indeed, ASWs are not the only gatekeepers in relation to section assessments; doctors, the police and even nearest relatives may be involved. This status as gatekeeper is created by statute and it will be helpful to explore this further - if somewhat schematically - as 'delegated authority'.

Social Problems: The ASW as gatekeeper is involved with a social problem (a matter of 'social concern'). Mental illness is not simply a health but also a social problem, evident from the wide variety of resources devoted to its alleviation, and a law permitting, under certain circumstances, compulsory admission. However, in what sense is it a social problem? Merton and Nisbett (1976) define social problems to exist 'where there is a sizeable discrepancy between what is and what ought to be'. If we take the state of mental health to be the 'ought' of this, then there is a significant proportion of the population at any one time in a state which they 'ought not' to be. Thus, 391 people per 100,000 population were admitted to mental hospitals in England in 1982 (DHSS, 1985). An even stronger 'ought not' is the combination of mental disorder with a 'health or safety' danger to the patient, or where 'protection of others' is required. Thus, 12,382 actions assessing compulsory admissions were taken by ASWs in 42 authorities during twelve months in 1985-6 (Bowl et al, 1987).

Merton and Nisbett (1976) also comment that 'whatever their origins, social problems are defined by their social consequences'. The personal consequences of mental illness can be considerable: distress to the patient, disruption of their lifestyle, and the effects on others can be marked. However, the nature of the collective response is a significant consequence: the development of extensive - if at times inadequate - resources, and the mobilisation of tens of thousands of people to deal both professionally and voluntarily with mental illness bears testimony to the social concern. In this respect we have some idea of the perceived magnitude of the problem, since this indicates not only the perceived *size* of the problem, but the *values* attached to it.

Norms and Social Problems: Mental illness, then, is a social problem. Classically, functionalist writers have divided social problems into two (Merton and Nisbett, 1976), social disorganisation and deviancy. Social disorganisation occurs when the society, or social system, fails to reach its own norm related objectives. If, for example, an objective is to achieve racial harmony, then persistent racial discrimination, with accompanying dissatisfaction, inequality and racial tension, represents social disorganisation. Race riots present this in a particularly vivid form.

Of more concern, when examining the role of gatekeeper, is deviant behaviour, of which mental illness is one type. When manifesting deviant behaviour an individual is transgressing or departing from norms. Thus Clinard, for example, defines deviant behaviour as 'essentially violations of certain types of group norms; a deviant act is behaviour which is proscribed in a certain way' (Clinard, 1968). Cohen states that 'deviant behaviour [is] behaviour which violates institutionalised expectations - that is expectations which are shared and recognised within a social system' (Cohen, 1950). Such behaviour is generally recognised in relation to the particular roles or statuses a person occupies, and which are socially assigned. Hence, for example, a child abuser may be a parent whose care of their children is seriously inadequate by comparison with standards expected of them as a child carer (i.e. in their role as parent). Parents are not expected to beat up their children, employees are not expected to defraud their employers and librarians are not expected to shout in the library.

As a social problem, then, mental illness (or mental disorder in general) is a form of deviance which is norm related. When a person displays signs and symptoms of mental illness they are contravening social norms. The identification of social problems in terms of the discrepancy 'between what is and what ought to be' involves an implicit appeal to the concept of norms. Norms are important as standards against which an individual can measure what should or should not occur. According to Gibbons and Jones (1975) they are generally defined by sociologists as guides to action designed to produce behavioural regularity in societies (or collectivities) on the part of groups and individuals.

> 'Whether inferred from behaviour or directly observed in some way, norms are thought of as rules or guides to behaviour that are internal."

In terms of social problems these are value related. The norms against which the problems are being measured are considered desirable and important. Hence, in the case of mental illness, behaviour manifesting mental health is considered desirable, while symptoms of mental illness are not desirable. The norms themselves may be codified or explicit or something which is implicit and 'taken for granted'. Examples of the former would include laws or criminal statute, while the latter might, for example, relate to standards of behaviour in the family or conduct of oneself with other people in everyday life.

These norms are not unproblematic: they may differ according to where you stand in society. In order to qualify as a social problem it is necessary either that there is a wide degree of agreement about the matter of concern, or that significant or powerful groups within the society agree about the issue. Hence many sociologists say "people", "many people", "the majority of people" or a "functionally significant set of people" must regard the situation as departing from the standard to qualify as a social problem. When social norms are a matter of overwhelming consensus, as with laws prohibiting murder, this is not problematic. However, in other cases, for example alcohol consumption or marijuhana smoking, consensus may not exist. Those occupying different positions in the social structure tend to have different and sometimes conflicting interests and values, even when they share other interests and values.

An important general point is that the ways in which norms relating to social problems that are defined by the state are perceived will depend on the stance of the observer (hence some people feel less comfortable than others about social work involvement in compulsory admissions). It is certainly the case that, as Merton and Nisbett (1976) comment, people occupying positions of power and authority carry more weight in deciding social policy and what constitutes significant departures from social norms. Hence the power relations and structure of society can affect the definition of social problems.

Notwithstanding this, both the state - which legislates and has enormous administrative power - and gatekeepers are critical in establishing norms against which the social problems may be defined. Where gatekeeping is involved, a complex relationship can be seen between the state and the gatekeeper. The state may be seen as broadly defining the area of concern - illness, murder, embezzlement, mental illness and so on - and at times the appropriate action to be taken. Thus criminal behaviour may provoke a range of penalties where conviction is achieved. However, the gatekeeping professional will frequently have a great deal of discretion in two respects: in applying the particular policies to individuals and in determining in detail the norms which relate to specific situations. The involvement of ASWs with mental illness, then, involves them both in a relationship with the state and a concern with the norms associated with mental health and illness.

Society and Social Action: The gatekeeping role of the ASW also reflects a 'social action' ethic in relation to mental illness. The social response to a particular problem depends to a great degree on the predominant ethic relating to it. At one extreme an attitude of fatalism can exist - a belief that situations are practically pre-ordained, and the outcome cannot be modified by foreknowledge or intervention. At the other extreme, the 'ethic of responsibility' characterises societies in which such intervention is widespread, and where most things are seen to be subject to human control (Mannheim, 1936; Weber, 1946).

In the first case there will be very little action to prevent or resolve social problems which will be regarded as inevitable. In the second, both prevention and resolution will be characteristic and a greater sense of social problems will exist alongside a desire to do something about them. Of course, these are extremes, and most states will attempt some intervention. However, in moving from a 'fatalist' to a 'responsible' standpoint, the need for intervention becomes a moral responsibility.

The circumstances relating to mental illness provide one such situation. Not only do the resources testify to the interventionist position, it is clearly related to moral obligation. Thus, for example, sectioning mentally ill persons on the grounds of their own 'health or safety' involves undertaking compulsory admissions in the person's own interests - it is what is good for them since they may become ill or injured or die.

Gatekeeping as Delegated Authority: The power of the ASWs as gatekeeper is closely tied up with their position in relation to the state. It involves the question of who it is that defines social problems. It should be noted immediately that the position of the state in identifying, defining and reacting to social problems is itself problematic, and perceptions of this depend on the theoretical commitment of the commentator. Whether a model is consensus, conflict or pluralist has a profound impact on perceptions of the legitimacy of state action involving issues of conflict, power and appropriate response (Strasser, 1976). However, as Davies (1985; 1981) points out, social workers act primarily as agents of the state - clearly the case with ASWs, who are directly empowered by the state - and it is the issue of their relationship to the state, rather than the legitimacy of state action, which is of concern here in understanding their gatekeeping role.

Individuals assessed for compulsory admission are socially problematic: the position of ASWs in dealing with this socially problematic area is based on powers conferred on them by the state, and expressed in statute. In essence this means that a particular group (ASWs) have been considered particularly competent to deal with that area, and also *trusted* to do so competently. This position, according to Wilding (1982), develops because of the importance of their work to society or to certain parts of it. Hence the police deal with criminality, doctors with ill health, and social workers with a variety of problems. The relationship has a number of elements:

1. It involves the notion that certain important parts of life are *properly delegated* to professionals as their responsibility: health is a matter for doctors, education for teachers, the care of certain need groups for social workers.

2. They develop a significant role as deliverers of key services, which means that government comes to depend on the professions in relation to their welfare commitments. This power reinforces the profession's ability, for the practice of particular activities, to be restricted to those with professional qualifications.

3. They tend to define the issue as a personal problem, susceptible to individual solutions by experts (which effectively de-politicises the social problem).

4. In dealing with these problems, the professions provide individual services in which external supervision is difficult, and routine standardised procedures are impossible. Again this is related to the personalised perception of problems, which emphasises the importance of individuals in the treatment.

The essence of the relationship to the state in legitimising their gatekeeping role, then, is the individualised perception of problems, the narrowing down of those competent to a selected group, and the claim of that group to particular competence. The devolution of this responsibility, however, can involve the exercise of power in certain circumstances. Hence doctors may diagnose someone as ill, allowing them access to the sick role and legitimate absence from work; police may arrest, and courts may remand someone into custody; and ASWs (with others) may admit some people against their will to mental hospital.

Gatekeepers as Rule Enforcers: How are we to consider this 'delegated authority' in relation to the particular issue of compulsory admissions? From what do ASWs *specifically* derive their authority?

When we consider the issue of compulsory admissions we immediately move into the arena of law. The immediate source of the power of the ASW - that which legitimates their role - is the law relating to compulsory admission, residing in the Mental Health Act. It is because they are empowered by the state, through the Mental Health Act, that ASWs may legitimately involve themselves in compulsory admissions. However, the Act itself leaves a great deal of room for interpretation. This room means that the gatekeepers involved - ASWs, doctors, the nearest relative and so on - are able to exercise a great deal of discretion, and hence power, in individual situations.

In order to explain how this is possible, we need to understand more about the two most significant elements of the situation, the law and mental health. Both of these may be understood in terms of rules (which give expression to the norms discussed earlier), for ASWs are best conceptualised, when making compulsory admission assessments, as rule enforcers.

The Law

H.L.A. Hart (1961) saw law in terms of rules. He identified a number of types of rules relating to law: primary and secondary rules, and rules of recognition, rules of change and rules of adjudication. It is the last of these - rules of adjudication - with which we are concerned. What are these? They are rules which empower individuals to make authoritative statements on the question of whether, on a particular occasion, a law has been broken. This is the kind of activity with which higher courts are often involved. It essentially involves interpreting particular laws to make clear, where there is some uncertainty, what that particular law means, or how it should be applied in specific circumstances.

A well-known example relates to the 1989 Dock Strike which arose following the repeal of the Act enforcing the Dock Labour scheme. The issue raised was whether the dock strike was political or merely an industrial dispute. If it were a political dispute it would have been illegal. The case went to the Law Lords where they decided that, despite its being a response to the Act's repeal, it was an industrial and *not* a political dispute. In circumstances where the law was insufficiently clear about what exactly constituted a political strike, they were able to use their discretion to make judgements where the precise interpretation of the law was not obvious.

Hart calls this domain of uncertainty within the law the 'open texture of law'. This uncertainty may surprise those who see laws as sets of rules which define, in a black and white way, what is and what is not allowed within the law. The problem is that, to a considerable degree, the law is concerned with generalities - general standards - which, as with the above example, do not always fit precisely with specific situations. Hence it was known that political strikes were illegal; what was problematic was whether or not the dockers' proposed actions *were* political.

The difficulty is that the law is predominantly concerned with *classes* of persons or acts: in this case it was the class of act which was or was not political. However, sometimes the sphere to be legally controlled may contain enormous variations from one case to another. This means that uniform rules which can be applied from one case to another cannot usefully be framed by legislators in advance. In these circumstances, interpretation is delegated to a rule making body, which will then fashion rules adapted to a *particular* situation. This is a major task of precedent in English law.

In the case of the Mental Health Act, both rules of adjudication and the open texture of law are significant. The act is concerned with general classes of persons (the mentally disordered) or a general class of conditions (mental disorder). Hence one decision to be made is whether or not the patient is suffering a mental disorder. The other relevant concepts of the 'Health or Safety of the Patient' or 'Protection of Other Persons' are very imprecise. Although legal precedent may *in principle* operate, there are no recent examples of such interpretation. Guidance may be obtained from the Mental Health Act Commission, which loosely acts as adjudicator (Mental Health Act Commission, 1987).

The imprecision of the phrases 'his own health or safety' or 'the protection of other persons' places them firmly within the open texture of law, and this gives ASWs and doctors a great deal of discretion to interpret the law in particular circumstances. The gatekeepers, therefore, exercise a great deal of power which goes with the discretionary interpretation of the law. Indeed, the patient's only defence against misuse of this power (apart from appeal to the Mental Health Review Tribunal) is the requirement, enshrined in Section 139, that the ASW (and doctors) should not act 'in bad faith' or 'without reasonable care', which are extremely vague. It is because of this 'open texture of law' that issues of civil rights are of such significance.

Residual Rule-Breaking

The second set of rules with which ASWs are concerned relates to mental disorder in general, and mental ill health in particular. The Act, as is well known, provides no definition of mental illness, which is therefore left to clinical judgement. This again leaves the professionals involved - particularly in the medical diagnosis - with a great deal of discretion. In order to understand this relationship between rules and mental illness it is useful to examine the work of Scheff (1984)

Scheff develops the concept of residual rules. He identifies two sets of rules, both of which relate to norms of behaviour.

1. Explicitly identified rules, which are rules involving matters such as crime and drunkenness. These are rules which people are prepared to state, or write down, explicitly. Hence one generally accepted rule of social behaviour is that individuals should not become drunk and disorderly. Contravening this rule is likely to invite disapproval, or even a night in the cells.

2. The second set of rules are residual rules of behaviour. These are not rules which are explicitly identified, but are taken for granted. They are the rules of social behaviour which separate out, broadly speaking, what is considered normal and what is considered 'odd' or 'strange'. These behaviours are considered odd or strange because they seem to most people to be incomprehensible - they do not seem to make any sense.

Scheff suggests that those actions or perceptions which are considered to be symptoms of mental illness are contraventions of these residual rules. Hence hallucinations, delusions, withdrawal or continual muttering manifested by individuals, and which appear incomprehensible to others, are examples of residual rule breaking. The person who is defined as mentally ill because they are suffering symptoms such as hallucinations or delusions may also be seen, from a different perspective, to be involved in residual rule breaking.

The concept of residual rule breaking is relevant, of course, to any one particular culture. It can, however, be of particular use to ASWs practising in contemporary Britain. Residual rules, which define the difference between normal and strange, odd or incomprehensible behaviour, are culture related. Hence, while they are important in any one particular culture, it is particularly important in a multi-cultural country like Britain. What may be considered perfectly normal in one culture may appear quite strange in another. Hence, a belief of being 'possessed by devils', a phenomena acceptable in some cultures, would generally be considered to be a delusion in late twentieth century Britain. However, praying would not in Britain be perceived as evidence of mental illness, while 'talking to spirits' might in other cultures be perceived to be perfectly sane.

The fine distinctions evident here show the complexity of residual rules, and recognition of such rule breaking is itself a complex process (Rack, 1982). Residual rule breaking is a concept which provides a useful link between mental illness and culture and, in addition to being important in itself, is a considerable aide to developing ethnically sensitive practice.

ASWs as gatekeepers are therefore involved in a process where a further set of rules is considered: residual rules, in the form of psychiatric symptomatology. Although four broad categories of mental disorder are identified in the Act (Section 1) - mental impairment, severe mental impairment, psychopathic disorder and mental illness - the last of these is not defined and is left to clinical judgement. In so doing the law leaves this matter to delegated experts who may then decide on an individual basis about the presence or absence of mental illness. The 'open texture of law', therefore, involves the ASW in a process where further decisions about rules are made: whether or not residual rules have been broken.

The Function of Gatekeepers

The ASW, then, as gatekeeper is concerned with social problems in a society which, in relation to mental health issues, may be described as manifesting an ethic of responsibility. They achieve their position through a relationship with the state which empowers them in certain specified areas, and they operate through the application of rules which allow them a great deal of discretion in decision-making.

As gatekeepers, ASWs may be seen as serving two functions:

1. They can provide access to an official identity - examples of which are criminal suspect, patient and so on. The identity is official insofar as those who bestow it are, through the law, acting as officials on behalf of the state.

2. They can provide access to resources, such as residential care, hospital or financial resources.

Very often, although not always, these two elements, identity and resources, are connected. Access to identity (illness) may give access to resources (hospital). This does not mean the person seeks such an identity - as is clearly the case when mental health admissions are compulsory - and it certainly does not mean the identity is complimentary. It may, as with some criminality and mental illness, be extremely stigmatising.

The basis of their gatekeeping power is the presumed expertise and impartiality of the relevant professionals. This emanates from what Parsons (1949) calls the 'primacy of cognitive rationality' through which the professions claim to know better than other people the nature of certain matters. Rationality and expertise are very difficult to challenge in a society which depends so heavily on them. Thus it is faith in knowledge and competence which gives the medical profession the power to deal with illness and, to a lesser degree, social workers the power to deal with delinquents; a faith that the knowledge exists or may be developed and applied to solve problems.

This is precisely the situation relating to compulsory admission. Indeed, the 'open texture of the law', the assessment of mental illness according to clinical judgement, and the vagueness of the health or safety of the patient or protection of others criteria, may all be related to the delegation of authority to perceived experts. A long formal training is required to acquire such expertise - note the additional ASW training in this context - which is explicitly to inculcate knowledge and implicitly to establish professional identity.

This relates to a second element: the professionals' right to define needs and problems which provide the necessary legitimation for their exercise of power and authority. Marshall (1963) sees, as a crucial element in the professionals' claim to a particular status, that he or she has the responsibility of giving the client what he *needs* rather than what he *wants*. The professional defines the client's problems for him rather than accepting his (the client's) prior definition, in so doing conferring an identity on him.

This process has been called by Berger (1977) 'cognitive imperialism'. As regards defining the situation, this means that every 'inhabitant' of a world has an immediate access to it which is superior to that of the 'non inhabitant'. The 'worlds' at issue here are the views of the professional and client. This refers to the superiority of the professionals' view over that of the client - or other lay people - which means that one element of the situation, the 'non inhabitants' ' view, may be neglected or ignored. This is clearly the case with compulsory admission assessments: it is the professionals who define the presence or absence of mental illness and who identify the health or safety of the patient, or protection of others, dangers (except when the nearest relative is involved). If disagreement occurs, it is their view, and not that of the patient, which will carry the day, as is intended by the Act. Indeed, their expertise is seen to give them just such a right.

This is clearly evident in a closely related area. Fennel conducted research on Mental Health Review Tribunals (before the 1983 Act) (Fennel, 1977). When the patient disagreed with the psychiatrist, or disputed the facts as stated by him, it was interpreted as part of his symptomatology unless the patient could find someone to substantiate his story. To a considerable extent, therefore, psychiatrists were able to 'explain away' patients' complaints.

This recognition of expertise is not problematic if, as most ASWs no doubt do, we accept the necessity for such expertise in making judgements. Some sociologists are, however, less happy. Wilding (1982), for example, points to the supposed narrowness of professional vision which, because welfare professionals deal with individuals, leads them to conceptualise problems in individual rather than structural terms. In the case of compulsory admissions, however, it is not simply professional ideology which may be individualistic. The functions the ASW carries out are defined by law, and their role, dealing with individuals, is entirely appropriate within the context of the law.

The other major power of gatekeepers is that of resource allocation. Professional power in resource use is often substantial, and may be exercised with few political or bureaucratic constraints. The extent of the power which lies in the hands of individual gatekeepers, however, will depend on individual circumstances. First, it involves whether or not they actually control the resources. A GP may wish an elderly person to enter local authority residential care, but they must approach others in the social services department first. A similar situation confronts the ASW in relation to hospital beds with compulsory admission - they must approach the psychiatrist (or theoretically the hospital managers) first. Second, the power may be shared: an individual social worker cannot unilaterally accept a child voluntarily into care; they must consult others, generally senior professionals. Likewise, the decision to section an individual, when it involves the ASW, is a joint one, also involving medical professionals.

Resources are broadly of two types. Self resources involves rationalising access to the professional himself. Thus, like doctors, social workers have considerable freedom in deciding how to use the resource of their own time, involving appointment systems, availability and so on. Because they find family and child care work more rewarding (as well as priorities arising from pressure of work), social workers give more time and attention, and hence resources, to this kind of work (Howe, 1986; Rees, 1978). With compulsory admissions this may involve deciding when to make the assessment, how long it should take, and who to interview (although, of course, the ASW is likely to be influenced by the situation and other professional personnel in their time use).

In addition to being 'gatekeeper to his own resources', ASWs are 'gatekeepers to other resources'. This may refer either to human or material resources. Thus the social worker may provide clients access to a home help or family aide, or a specialist in a particular area of work who may be able to help them further. The ASW does this, when assessing for compulsory admission, in providing access - however unwilling the patient is to accept - to the human resources of medical, nursing and other paramedical staff. Alternatively, the resources may be material. Social workers can commit substantial amounts of departmental resources; their interpretation of a care order can commit many thousands of pounds of resources over many years, or no resources at all. This position is similar to that of the ASW when considering hospital admission; he is in effect committing expensive and extensive resources to the patient, or looking for alternatives (perhaps hostel accommodation, or nothing at all, depending on the decision made, jointly with doctors).

Civil Rights and the Nearest Relative: Although, of course, all these elements hold true for the ASW as gatekeeper, the role of the ASW as applicant may be taken by the nearest relative. This reflects an ambivalence within the Act about professional authority and power. On the one hand, it requires ASWs to possess 'appropriate competence'; on the other, the nearest relative may carry out their role. If sections were *always* undertaken by ASWs and doctors (they are anyway 90 per cent of the time) this would mean authority and power would be exclusively in professional hands. However, it will be strongly argued on the basis of this research that the position of the nearest relative is anomalous, that assessment of the health or safety of the patient or protection of others criteria is complex, requiring the development of expertise the nearest relative cannot possess, and that as a result the civil rights of the patient are better protected by the ASW.

Civil rights, as considered in this study, involve two elements. First, they involve the accurate and appropriate application of the law. Thus, for example, a patient should not be admitted under Sections 2, 3, or 4 unless they are believed, in good faith, to suffer a mental disorder; or admitted under Section 4 unless such admission is of 'urgent necessity' and complying with Section 2 would cause 'undesirable delay'. Second, assessment should take account of justice: the interpretation of which has been equal treatment for equals, according to relevant criteria. Essentially this means that if the ASW encounters two identical situations the outcome should be identical. It should not be the case that one patient is compulsorily admitted and the other is not hospitalised. However, the vagueness of the health or safety of the patient or protection of others criteria reflecting the 'open texture of law' suggests that such consistency should be demonstrated to exist rather than taken for granted. Given the number of ASWs involved in sections, such consistency is far from certain.

The ASW as Gatekeeper: Further Theoretical Issues

Civil rights are not, in practice, simply a matter of justice and appropriate application of rules. They occur in a social context, are applied by human beings, and are subject to the vagaries inevitable when humans are involved. Some issues, therefore, relating to the gatekeeping role require further consideration.

First, according to Friedson (1973), illness - whether physical or mental - is not simply a biophysical state, but a social state, bound up with people's beliefs, evaluations and actions. The former element, which is often referred to as a disease, involves abnormalities in the biological functioning of the human body which possess a biological reality independent of the way people think about them (for example, a broken leg). However, it is also a social state, because central to the notion of illness is a set of norms about health, normality and the 'way things should be' involving judgements about valued and not valued states; illness represents some deviation from a desirable state of affairs (health), and hence is connected to perceptions of what is or is not valued.

The doctor is highly significant in the process of illness definition. When in pain or unable to walk or unusually tired, a person will consult their doctors who will pronounce the person's deviance from normal functioning by giving a medical name to the condition (diagnosis). The person will be called 'ill' and a number of social consequences will follow, such as being relieved of normal expectations and duties (such as working), being given the appropriate medical care and so on.

The ill person effectively takes on a social role - the 'sick role' - to which the doctor gives him access. At the centre of this is the notion that there is agreement about what constitutes normal and abnormal functioning for which the doctor becomes the authority. The particular consequences accompanying this state - the need for treatment - depend on constructing the state as an illness, and ascribing an appropriate social role. In a sense, therefore, and without adopting an anti-psychiatric stance, all doctors may be seen as 'moral entrepreneurs' (or at least 'moral arbiters'), and ASWs when closely involved in the same process - as with compulsory admissions - may be identified similarly.

Szasz (1961) would take this issue further. He distinguishes between physical illness, which he considers legitimately the concern of medicine, and mental illness, where the term 'illness' is purely a metaphor for problems of living. However, using this term has consequences because it brings it within the boundaries of medicine. Unlike Friedson, he suggests that physical illness involves a biological 'value free' process, but that mental health - concerned with the control of behaviour, perceptions and moods - is involved with the enforcement of morals.

Although, with Friedson, we may dispute this, Szasz is correct to assert that mental health, unlike (generally) physical medicine, does not always require the consent of the subject for treatment to occur. Indeed, this is the very essence of compulsory admissions, that someone is admitted against their will to hospital for assessment, treatment or both (under Sections 2, 3 or 4). In this respect, Szasz's concern for liberty can be separated, in part, from his assertion that mental illness is a euphemism for 'problems of living'. Of course, Section 131 allows for informal admission to hospital which frequently occurs as an alternative to compulsory admission. However, he suggests that there is no such thing as 'informal' admission when the only alternative is compulsory admission, for if you do not go in informally you will be sectioned (compulsorily admitted) anyway. In such cases you are not at liberty to choose *not* to enter hospital, just the status under which you will be hospitalised (cf. Bowl, Barnes and Fisher, 1987). This means that once the decision to admit has been taken by the professionals the patient is deprived of his freedom, regardless of his wishes.

Scheff (1984) identifies a tendency in medicine towards a 'presumption of illness' which is particularly problematic in conjunction with the previous point. It is a cultural norm (of the occupation) and like other cultural norms is one that is not examined in a day-to-day context, but is one that in medicine 'goes without saying'. It arises because of the seriousness of the conditions with which doctors deal and the consequences of getting it wrong. If a doctor diagnoses cancer wrongly (i.e. he diagnoses it as present when it is, in fact, absent), there are unlikely to be any long term consequences, at least in physical terms (the emotional impact of such a misdiagnosis could be very great). If, however, a doctor fails to diagnose cancer when it is, in fact, present, this could lead to a serious deterioration in the patient and, if the mistake remained undiscovered for long enough, quite possibly death.

Doctors are inevitably involved in such difficult decisions, and the 'presumption of illness' means that when in doubt they will tend to diagnose illness rather than health, thus erring on the side of safety. This may be fine, Scheff thinks, with physical disorder, but such labelling could do 'untold damage' to someone diagnosed mentally ill. It is both stigmatising, he thinks, and likely to create a situation in which the person takes on the identity of a mentally ill person, perceiving themselves as mentally ill in a form of 'secondary deviance'. Again, we do not have to accept Scheff's labelling theory (of mental illness being solely the social creation of professional labellers) to recognise that the 'presumption of illness' could lead to unnecessary loss of liberty in relation to compulsory admissions (cf. Bean, 1980).

The point is further emphasised if, in addition to Scheff's ideas, we introduce a concomitant notion of the 'presumption of risk' in relation to the criteria of the 'health or safety of the patient' and 'protection of other persons'. This would reflect a similar dilemma to that of the doctor utilising the 'presumption of illness'. The consequences of failing to recognise significant risk when it is present would be considered far worse than the consequences of identifying risk where it is not in fact present. Hence, the ASW would, when making this presumption, have a tendency to view the mentally ill person as inherently risky - perhaps because of perceived unpredictability - even when the evidence for this might appear slim.

The link between the 'presumption of illness' and civil rights of the patient can be made through Bean's (1980) distinction between legal versus treatment orientations. Legalism shows itself whenever there is a concern to act according to the rule of law. The main assumption about legalism is that no one should be confined to any institution without specific legal safeguards, in particular that the machinery and personnel of the law - the courts and magistrates - should have a critical part to play. An obvious example of this in a social work context is the compulsory reception into care of children, which can only take place based on the agreement of magistrates and courts. The treatment approach emphasises that the person's need for treatment *overrides* his legal right to be represented by counsel and appear in court. In such cases the decisions are made purely by the authorised professionals; in the case of the Mental Health Act primarily by doctors and approved social workers, although the nearest relative may be the applicant instead of the ASW. The 1959 Act represented a drift from legalism, largely maintained in the 1983 Act, although legalism does appear after admission in the form of the patient's right to be told of his rights, his right to appeal to the Mental Health Review Tribunal, and his right to request legal aid on appeal.

When a treatment approach predominates, as in the 1983 Act, the scope for making decisions purely on the basis of illness is more evident. This is more serious when the 'presumption of illness' approach operates. Although Bean does not accept that psychiatrists operate this presumption, he suggests that the 1959 Act vested too much power in doctors, and it did so because of the excessive emphasis on the treatment needs of the patient to the detriment of a recourse to legal institutions and representation. The danger resided in therapeutic legal rules adopted by psychiatrists which allowed for a form of discretionary justice dispensed in private by experts. The psychiatrists, trained in medicine, were concerned primarily about the illness and treatment requirements of their patients. This led to an emphasis on therapeutic aims to the detriment of legal rules. Rules which aided therapeutic aims were emphasised, those which did not were regarded with suspicion. This could lead, in some circumstances, to patients being compulsorily admitted in contravention of the spirit and even the letter of the law, a situation which would have been less likely had recourse to legal institutions and personnel first been necessary.

Finally, the 'knowledge orientation' of involved professionals is significant. Clearly, as we have argued, the health or safety of the patient and protection of other persons criteria involve social considerations, in the sense that they are part of a particular social problem, they involve reference to implicit or explicit norms of behaviour, they relate frequently to social relationships (such as protecting others from the patient) and they are invoked as part of a social process of assessing for compulsory admission. The social context is further emphasised by the known impact of social factors on the aetiology, progress and prognosis of mental illness.

Huntington (1981) argues that the knowledge base of medicine tends towards the 'biophysical' and of social work towards the 'psychosocial'. The tendency towards the biophysical is evident in the earlier discussion about the nature of illness, in which medicine emphasises the objective physiological characteristics without reference to social norms or social context. Social workers, on the other hand, have a training which immerses them in the psychosocial context of their clients. Hence they will tend to place clients in their social context, examine the cause and process of their problems in terms of psychosocial factors, and attempt to identify the meaning to clients of the particular circumstances in which they find themselves.

Bean (1980) indicates that their psychiatric training leads psychiatrists to reinterpret social factors in terms of psychiatric symptoms, a reflection of their professional assumptions and concerns. The orientation of professionals might be expected to influence the relative importance ascribed by them to mental disorder, one of the criteria for compulsory admission, *versus* the criteria of the health or safety of the patient and protection of other persons. The latter are frequently more social in orientation, for they can involve explicit reference to the interaction of the patient with other people as well as his own *behaviour* which has implications for his health or safety. If the emphasis of the assessment is strongly placed on the mental disorder element, we might expect to find some difficulty in accounting for compulsory admissions in terms of the health or safety of the patient or protection of other persons or some obscuring of this dimension.

We have now some awareness of the major dimensions of the analysis of the role of the ASW as gatekeeper. They are concerned with mental illness (and compulsory admissions in particular) not because it is a health problem - although this is how it is defined - but because it is a *social problem*, a situation which contrasts with that of doctors whose authority arises specifically because of their expertise in diagnosing health and illness. The ASW involvement also derives from their concern with social norms, and as such they both assess rule contravention and are rule enforcers. Their authority derives from statute.

At this stage we cannot elucidate their role as gatekeepers any further. However, a number of further factors have been identified whose influence needs to be considered when examining the ASW as gatekeeper and rule enforcer, and which may affect the civil rights of people assessed for compulsory admission. The analysis of the criteria of health or safety of the patient and protection of other persons, therefore, must display awareness of the value positions adopted by ASWs; the extent to which a 'presumption of risk' exists; the relationship between perception of illness and the nature and perception of risk; the relative importance of therapeutic issues and adherence to rules; and the clarity with which the health or safety of the patient and protection of other persons issues are formulated.

The Assessment of Risk: A Framework for Analysis

The assessment of risk is implicit in the health or safety of the patient or protection of others criteria. Fisher, Newton and Sainsbury (1984) comment that, in contrast with child care, social workers did not, under the 1959 Act, attempt to evaluate risk against 'normal' risk taking in the community. Bean (1980) used the concept of danger to indicate the likelihood of compulsory admission. However, he concentrated primarily on psychiatrists, not social workers, and used predefined ratings rather than developing categories from the professionals' own accounts. Risk assessment is a central aspect of social work practice. Indeed, Brearley (1982) suggests most social work involves some element of risk. Certainly risk is involved in many aspects of child care, mental health and elderly work.

The interpretation of the practical implementation of health or safety of the patient or protection of others criteria requires the development of an appropriate conceptual framework. This relies critically on the concept of risk. Brearley provides a particularly helpful starting point. His central concern is to 'unpack' the concept of risk, thus providing concepts and a framework for analysis of use to social work. It involves issues like harm, uncertainty, probability and prediction, but the most central are risk itself, hazard, and danger.

Risk, according to Brearley, 'refers to the relative variations in possible loss outcomes' where a 'loss outcome' refers, for example, to harm to the subject. All situations, he suggests, have some element of risk and uncertainty, even walking down the street. Hence risk does not simply involve criteria of 'risk versus no risk' but discriminating the acceptable from the unacceptable. Rowe (1977) suggests a process:

    1.   Establishing a risk referent level (i.e. acceptable risk).

    2.   Determining the level of risk (in a proposed action).

3. Comparing the risk with the referent.

4. Risk aversive action.

Hazard, Brearley states, 'refers to any existing factor - an action, event, situation or entity - which introduces the probability of an undesirable outcome'. It is clearly related to risk, insofar as each additional hazard creates a new possibility for a 'loss outcome'. Examining hazard involves identifying what the person is exposed to, what are the possible adverse effects, and *how much* adverse effects are likely to occur (Lowrence, 1976).

Danger is the third element, and Brearley uses it as a term to cover the various concepts of 'negative outcome', 'feared loss', or 'unpleasant circumstances'. Danger is related to hazard as its possible end product: if a hazard exists, the danger represents the feared outcome which *becomes a possibility* in the face of the hazard. However, a further element of danger is that it is forward looking - it is an outcome which may happen at some future time. In this it differs from *damage,* which is something that is current or has already occurred. In this respect, danger represents some future feared damage.

Clearly, these three concepts - danger, hazard and risk - are closely interconnected. They possess common elements: they are future looking rather than focussed on current happenings (although current occurrences may provide evidence of risk); they involve an element of probability - we cannot be sure, but only estimate, the likelihood of a feared outcome; finally, they involve an element of prediction - when we assess risk we are making some prediction, no matter how tentative, of likely outcome.

Assessment and Use of Evidence

Rational assessment, by definition, involves giving reasons for the conclusion reached, and risk is no different in this respect. This is closely associated with the nature and use of evidence collected in the assessment process. Haines (1975) suggests the assessment task is:

> 'to gather together as much information as possible and form some opinion of its meaning for the client and its implications for action.'

It is centrally concerned, for Haines, with accumulating facts and identifying feelings from the client, family and environment, and weighing the importance of these, and their significance for the client, before coming to some conclusion.

However, this is not a simple neutral activity. We would be completely overwhelmed if we simply examined the 'facts of the matter' since in any situation there are innumerable factors to consider. We need, in fact, some mechanism by which we can identify which factors are *relevant* to our assessment, and also the relative *importance* we may ascribe to each of these (Sheppard, 1984). We need, in short, to know what to look at and how to interpret it. In this respect, our assessment is 'theory laden' (Howe, 1987) and this allows us to ascribe meaning to the situation.

Such 'signposts' are critical for compulsory admissions. The ASW is confronted with the immediate problem; what is happening here? They may have little previous knowledge of the patient; they may have information from various quarters; and they have to observe the patient. It is necessary to create a meaningful picture from the disparate pieces of information. There are, though, further problems. Mental illness is a controversial concept, and the ASW and doctors may at times find themselves holding different perspectives. Furthermore, the situation is sometimes a crisis; the circumstances may be dangerous, pressure may be exerted by doctors, friends or relatives, and decisions may have to be taken quickly. In a fraught situation, the ASW will need ways of interpreting evidence in order to make a meaningful assessment.

Values and the Threshold of Risk

A useful concept when analysing compulsory admission is that of the 'threshold of risk'. By this I mean the threshold beyond which patients are considered to be of sufficient risk to be compulsorily admitted . This threshold is incorrigibly normative. Some *types* of risk are acceptable - we do not stop someone from entering the dangerous sport of Grand Prix racing. Others are not - young children are not expected to be left alone in the house. Equally, some *levels* of risk are acceptable while others are not.

The acceptable level of risk will vary according to values. If your main value is 'respect for life' you may insist an elderly person at risk enters residential care. If it is 'respect for persons' you may wish to allow them to stay at home - if that is their wish - regardless of risk (always assuming you have the requisite power). This value clash underlies many of the disputes between doctors and social workers in this area.

These factors come together to form a framework through which the health or safety of the patient or protection of others may be analysed:

Nature of danger)	
To whom the threat exists)	
Nature of hazard)	Health or safety of
Level of risk)	patient and/or
Evidence provided)	protection of others
Threshold of risk)	

Area and Method

The core of this study is the examination of 120 referrals for assessment for compulsory admission. These referrals were made to a Mental Health Advice Centre over a one year period from 1 December 1987 to 31 November 1988 inclusive. They originated from a variety of sources including GPs, the police, psychiatrists and relatives of the patients, and they were assessed by nine approved social workers. Six of these ASWs were based in a health setting, while the other three were based in area teams, but undertook regular 'duty' periods at the Centre.

The Centre is situated in a central location in an urban setting. The city has a population of about a quarter of a million, although it has a very small ethnic minority population. This is unfortunate in view of the impact of ethnicity, already discussed, on referral and decision to admit, and it means the study is not representative of areas with significant ethnic minority populations. However, it does possess the advantage that, because race issues do not appear, the decision to admit will not have been affected by overt or covert racism. Hence, when examining the criteria of health or safety of the patient or protection of others, the clarity of the ASWs' accounts will not have been affected by a desire to conceal racist elements.

The Centre had been in existence for ten years before the research began and was therefore already well established as a focus for referral. Its personnel primarily involve social workers and community psychiatric nurses, and referrals are received by workers who are on duty each day. Compulsory admission assessments form one part of their work, which also involves counselling, psychiatric assessment and, at times, crisis intervention. The majority of referrals for compulsory admission assessments in the city are received by the Centre rather than through the area teams. In relation to these assessments, therefore, three ASWs based in area teams regularly provide the social work input with section assessments originating from referrals received by the Centre.

The research was based mainly on semi-structured interviews undertaken with the ASWs following each individual referral. The interview schedule was developed with the ASWs during a pilot period, although it was considerably helped by the fact that the author is himself an ASW and has undertaken many compulsory admission assessments. It can at times be a problem getting access to an organisation and its workers, both because of the time the research takes and a fear of possible results. In fact the study benefited from the immediate co-operation of the ASWs. There were already strong links with the author through education and training and the social workers were very interested in standards of practice and saw this as an opportunity for closer examination of their work.

The schedule was based around two elements: a structured part, which recorded information on the referrer, the request, diagnosis and outcome; and a semi-structured part. This latter part focussed centrally on the process of assessment, how the situation was defined, and the reasons the ASWs gave for the action they took. It was based around a few key questions:

> What were the social circumstances which led to referral?

> What in detail were the problems of health or safety for the patient? Or (for the protection of others) who needed protecting and from what did they need protecting?

> Further information was also collected on why particular sections were chosen, why informal admission was not made,and ,where admission was refused, the reason for this. Additionally, the interview sought to establish the degree of agreement or disagreement between the ASWs and doctors in individual assessment. A further question, therefore, of importance in relevant cases was:

> If disagreement occurred between the professionals, what were the alternative positions adopted?

The approach adopted, then, was to obtain accounts from the ASWs of the process of intervention. This is quite different, for example, from the approach Bean (1980) made which emphasised direct observation as well as structured and semi-structured questionnaires. However, if our central question is how did the ASWs interpret in practice the (loose) criteria of health or safety of the patient or protection of other persons, it is necessary for them to report what it was *they* thought they were doing. There is little to be gained in this respect from direct observation. Burgess (1984) comments that:

> 'The value of being an observer lies in the opportunity that is available to collect rich detailed data based in natural settings.'

This would give us direct access to what in fact ASWs actually did. However, our concern is not so much this - although interesting in itself - as how they perceived or accounted for what they were doing; that is how they saw themselves to be interpreting the relevant legislation. This is best achieved by asking ASWs to say what they thought they were doing. Indeed, it is possible that direct observation could affect both the questioning and the way questions were answered, insofar as the ASWs may take for granted the interviewer's acquaintance with the situation in giving their answers.

Likewise, agency records, although interesting, were not appropriate sources of information. Their main problem is that they are used for entirely different purposes from the research. This could lead to a number of difficulties: they may be incomplete, or written some considerable time after the event; the accuracy of the information is inevitably questionable since they were not originally written for subsequent research; the terms may be vague and imprecise; and the issues they address may have little to do with the concerns of the research. There were, in fact, great variations in the ways individual ASWs wrote about admission, and the length of their reports. Some made detailed comments on the referral, who was involved and what happened; others would simply write, for example, 'Section 3 completed'.

Fully structured questionnaires would, of course, have been entirely inappropriate in attempting to identify the types of circumstances which ASWs considered to fit the criteria of the health or safety of the patient or the protection of other persons since by creating arbitrary categories the questionnaires would anticipate what the research sought to discover. Before the research began we were in no position to develop such categories without imposing an external set of criteria upon the ASWs. As Phillips (1983) points out, where knowledge is thin, small scale qualitative research can be more useful, whereas quantitative methods, often based on the developments of qualitative research, may be more appropriate in refining hypotheses.

The semi-structured interviews, however, possessed a number of advantages. They provided the opportunity for giving a detailed insight into particular issues based on the answers the ASWs gave. They gave the ASWs an opportunity to give reasons for the answers they gave, to elucidate them or to qualify them as appropriate. They allowed the ASWs to state, in their own terms, what they thought was going on and hence worked within their perspective or frame of reference. Finally, interviews can only be fully structured if the range of alternative answers is known beforehand, which in this case it was the purpose of the research to establish.

It was necessary to interview the ASWs in order to obtain the relevant information. If, for example, they were left with forms to fill out they may easily have ended up like case records - if, indeed, they were filled in at all - thus defeating the purpose of the project. The order of the questions asked is an important consideration. Akroyd and Hughes (1981) comment that:

> 'It could be that a question asked early in an interview affects answers to subsequent questions, and if this order were to be altered in any way it becomes difficult to detect the effect this may have on replies.'

These considerations were reflected in the interviews with the ASWs. Thus questions were consistently asked in the same order. However, the order itself was designed to reflect the most appropriate means for information gathering. Thus the first question sought to obtain a general description of the social circumstances of the patient, which provided a context against which the issues of health or safety of the patient or protection of others could be considered. From there the choice of section, the reasons, where relevant, for not admitting, and any disagreements with doctors were considered.

The nature of the information sought created particular problems in the interview process. In seeking to establish the way in which the health or safety or protection of others criteria were interpreted in practice it was necessary to be sure, as far as possible, that in replying to the relevant questions the ASW had done justice to their reasons for admitting. If, therefore, the answer was brief, there would be a need to explore further to discover whether that brevity reflected their reasoning or whether in fact their reasons were more complex or detailed and they had simply failed to state them adequately. However, it was also necessary to avoid 'leading' the ASW and, in particular, to import an inappropriate clarity into their assessments by implying, through the questions, distinctions between hazards, dangers and risk which they did not in fact make in practice. This may have been all too easy when attempting to probe further into the reasons for admission.

The problem, therefore, involved two issues: how, where relevant, to elicit more information from the ASW, but also when to stop. This was tackled by adopting a consistent approach to all the interviews. If the initial answer made by the ASW to the question relating to the health or safety of the patient or protection of others was brief they would simply be asked to amplify their statement. This would allow them to elucidate in more detail the way they saw themselves to be acting. However, this was done only once: if little extra information was obtained there was no further attempt to obtain information. Asking the ASW to 'amplify' their original statement, while inviting more detail, did not lead them in any direction as may have occurred if further questions had been asked in a flexible response to the initial statements. Much of the concern was with the ASWs' conceptual clarity rather than merely comprehensiveness of information. Hence this approach would not, simply by obtaining greater detail, be less likely to lead to greater conceptual clarity than the ASW in fact used when making the assessment. Equally, however, it would not be expected to conceal conceptual clarity where it did in fact exist. It is, of course, not possible to state conclusively that the accounts given by ASWs were unaffected by this approach to questioning. The approach did nonetheless attempt to take into account some of the difficulties. Overall, however, this did not present too great a problem; the ASWs were generally able to give fairly clear accounts of their actions without the need for further requests for information. This may well have reflected the interest and enthusiasm with which the ASWs approached the research, which will have made them concerned to provide adequate information.

The second dimension of analysis, additional to the conceptual clarity with which they undertook assessment, was the classification of the circumstances ASWs considered to be a threat to a patient's health or safety or the protection of other persons. This is a painstaking task, and was developed through the examination of the statements made by the ASWs. This entailed reading and re-reading the ASW accounts in order to be satisfied that the answers were categorised correctly. Initial classification was inevitably provisional, and refinement occurred as the interviews were re-examined.

The interviews with ASWs, from which this information was obtained, were always conducted during the week following the section assessment and, as a result, there was no problem of recall. The interviews generally lasted about fifteen to twenty minutes, although some lasted longer - the longest being 25 minutes. There was a great variation in the number of referrals from week to week; during some weeks no referrals were received, while the maximum received in any one week was seven. The pressure for information collection varied accordingly. However, both the ASWs and interviewer were at pains to ensure the success of the project, and the ASWs always responded positively to requests for interviews. This was considerably helped by the proximity of the Centre to the author's place of work. Hence it was easy to get to the Centre regularly and at relatively short notice. The ASWs, as a matter of course, filled in blue referral forms when section assessments were undertaken. These were collected and the previous week's assessments were made available to the author on the Monday. From this, both the person referred and the ASW undertaking the assessment were noted. The ASWs undertaking the assessments were then contacted and arrangements were made to interview them before the end of the week. There was some flexibility on both the part of the ASW and the author, and meetings occasionally had to be postponed because of an unexpected emergency. However, even in these cases, the interview always occurred before the end of the working week. This was, of course, important to ensure there was no problem of recall.

The outcome of these assessments was as follows:

Section 2: 34 cases
Section 3: 35 cases
Section 4: 1 case
Informal (compulsory) (If patient had refused admission they would have been sectioned): 20 cases
Other informal: 4 cases
No admission: 26 cases

TOTAL: 120 cases

Compared with the figures of Bowl et al (1987), which cover a wide number of authorities, considerably fewer patients were admitted under Section 4 (less than one per cent compared with 15.1 per cent). This was largely because of the ready availability of Approved Doctors to those working at the Centre. However, the number of informal admissions, which with patient refusal would have been compulsory, as with the national figures, is noticeably high. As Szasz points out, these patients are, in effect, deprived of their liberty because they have no choice about *whether or not* to enter hospital, just the status under which they go. Most practitioners would, however, consider informal admission less draconian and preferable where possible to compulsory admission. Certainly, Section 131 of the Act encourages informal admission where possible and appropriate. As well as those patients who were sectioned, this analysis includes patients who were informally admitted but who would have been sectioned had they not agreed to admission. In these cases the ASW will have been satisfied that the health or safety of the patient or protection of others criteria were fulfilled (because they would have admitted them compulsorily had they not agreed).

PART TWO

ASSESSMENT FOR COMPULSORY ADMISSIONS BY ASWs

The 1983 Act places the ASW in an independent position when assessing for compulsory admission. However, the necessary presence of at least one medical practitioner means that this decision is not made *alone*. Their involvement means that consultation between ASW and doctors will invariably occur, and frequently - though not always - collaborative joint visits will take place. This means that the ASW's perceptions are likely to be influenced by those of the doctors even when they disagree, since in disagreeing they will usually have to marshall their arguments to provide - for themselves at least - a convincing case.

However, the judgement of the ASW will inevitably be influenced by the clarity with which they undertake their assessment. Where both professions share the same assumptions they may often share the same judgements, without subjecting those assumptions to the scrutiny they would have attracted if they were not shared. Hence it would be a mistake to *assume* clarity of analysis without subjecting the *actual behaviour* of ASWs to close examination. This is the central concern of this chapter.

Dangers and Hazards

Hazards are factors which introduce the possibility of an undesirable outcome and dangers are the feared outcome. This difference may be illustrated by a simple example:

> 'watch out for the banana skin on the pavement, for you may slip and hurt yourself (if you walk on it)'.

Here the danger is that you may 'slip and hurt yourself' and the hazard is the banana skin.

An original intention of the research was to elucidate the nature of both dangers and hazards in ASWs' accounts. However, in many cases the ASWs' accounts, interestingly, reveal them less concerned with dangers than hazards: instead of indicating clearly the likely outcome if the patient were not admitted, they left this implicit in their account. This would be evident, extending our example, in the statement: 'Watch out, there is a banana skin on the pavement', or simply, 'There is a banana skin on the pavement'.

Such statements are less precise because we do not state *why* the hazard is significant: there is no indication of the danger that you might hurt yourself. In the context of compulsory admissions such lack of precision can have implications in terms of less clarity about the purpose of admission.

Where the danger is clearly indicated (48 cases). In these cases the hazard was also identified. One schizophrenic* man, for example, persecuted by thoughts that he would kill children, had been wandering around for days and had been picked up by the police. The ASW comments that:

> 'He was at great risk because of his slashed wrists which were getting infected. He was saying he would wander off if he was allowed, yet the slashes were so bad they (the doctors) could not stitch them.'

Clearly there was an implicit health danger - that his wounds might become infected while the hazard was that, having slashed his wrists, he might not get the medical attention he required (by wandering off). An additional implicit danger was that he would attempt suicide by again slashing his wrists.

Another example from this group was of a schizophrenic woman. She had stopped taking medication, was considered 'extremely volatile, restless and unreasonable'. She was also accusing her husband of having affairs. The ASW commented that:

> 'Although she was eating and drinking, it was irregular. Also she wasn't sleeping, and because she was too restless she was becoming exhausted. The section was for her health rather than her safety.'

---

* Throughout this study, wherever a patient is described as suffering a particular illness, this reflects the assessment of the ASW.

A third case was of a manic woman, whom the ASW described as:

> 'Rushing all over the place without thinking what she was doing. She wasn't sleeping or even stopping to take breath.....if she kept up at that rate she'd eventually collapse of fatigue.'

In both these cases the danger was clear: exhaustion or collapse, as was the hazard - lack of food, sleeplessness, and restlessness or hyperactive behaviour. The presence of the hazard in the ASW's accounts indicating the danger is not perhaps surprising: although it is possible in principle to mention the danger alone in order to explain *why* the danger was present it was necessary to refer to the hazard. Any meaningful account of danger, therefore, requires a hazard reference.

Where hazard is indicated and the danger is obvious (30 cases). The reverse is not, however, the case. In many of their accounts, the ASWs mentioned only the hazard without an explicit reference to danger. However, despite this, in some circumstances the danger, although implicit, was nonetheless clear. One retired man - morbidly jealous of his wife - was following her around, closely examining various items of her clothing. He was, commented the ASW:

> 'becoming more aggressive and waving a knife at her'.

Although only 'waving', the implication was clear: given his fixed and obsessive jealousy this could well become direct knife threats placing her in danger of injury or death.

Another woman, considered to be manic, was found by the police lying in the middle of the road in a 'completely incoherent state'. The ASW commented that she was:

> 'lying down in the middle of the road, listening to her son in Australia. She had no concept of the danger'.

Although unstated, the danger was obvious - that she might be injured or killed by passing traffic, or that others might be when drivers tried to avoid her.

Another case, also of a manic woman, suggested, without stating, a similar danger. She was very agitated, and became abusive. She was insisting on wandering around wherever she wished, which included the main road, but 'she had completely lost any road sense' and was likely to wander onto the road without any prior warning and whenever she felt like it. Although again unstated, the danger was obvious.

Where hazard is indicated, but the danger is unclear (20 cases).* Not all the cases where the hazard only was mentioned had an obvious danger. One single schizophrenic woman who lived on her own, and whose electricity had been cut off three months previously, had not drawn any social security benefit 'for some time', although she did have some money in the house. The ASW's concern was that:

> 'she had no electricity. She couldn't cook and wouldn't have any lighting at night'.

She also noted the woman had no friends to help her. The danger to this woman, from this account, is unclear. Is it the fear that her health might deteriorate from lack of cooked food? Or that she might fall over and hurt herself in the dark? If so, how had she managed these last three months? Likewise, did it matter that she had no friends if she had managed quite well without them? Because the danger is not identified we - and quite possibly the ASW - are left unsure of the threat to her health or safety.

Likewise a schizophrenic man who had left his home at night, taking some money with him, was considered at risk. Although not aggressive, the ASW worried that:

> 'he had been wandering the streets at night and the early hours of the morning, and he was quite dishevelled. He was not really rational'

There is perhaps more cause for concern here, but the danger is not clearly indicated. Was it that he might be attacked and hurt? Possibly robbed? That he might suffer exposure (although it was the middle of summer)? Or that traffic might hit and injure him? We are left to speculate.

---

* When the relevant figures are added together, they will total at times above 90 (the total number of sections and relevant informal admissions). This is because on occasion both the health or safety *and* protection of others was at issue. In some cases both criteria yielded the same approach (e.g. clearly identifying danger). In a few, however, they did not. Where 'crossover' occurred this always involved a combination of 'danger clearly indicated' and 'hazard indicated and danger obvious'. The 'hazard indicated - danger unclear' category was never combined with another category in an individual case.

Another schizophrenic woman believed she was the Queen, which her family was not keen to accept. She became quarrelsome with her family and neighbours who said it was nonsense, and became more socially isolated from them. When asked about the risk, the ASW said:

> 'It's difficult to say. She was causing problems with her neighbours because of the bit about the Queen, and she was beginning to neglect herself a bit.'

Many of this group referred to inadequate food intake. In addition to the first example, a schizophrenic man was sectioned because he had stopped eating, although it was not clear for how long, and he had not visibly lost weight. Another woman whose mental disorder was unclear 'wasn't eating properly', and may have been at risk 'if the situation had continued'. But she was being supported by her husband and was eating under his supervision. There were common factors in these and other cases: there was no indication of how long the patient had not eaten, or how long before health deterioration would occur, or if they would eat when hungry enough, or whether they might eat properly, if *appropriate* supports were given.

Two issues arise from this. 'Not eating' may - in some cases - have been an excuse for incarceration. This does not mean that sections were carried out in bad faith - a means for deliberately admitting people without good reason - but rather that lack of clarity led to 'admission by default'. Second, risk taking appears thereby to have been reduced in the way suggested by Fisher et al (1984). However, this is misleading. Closer examination suggests that, rather than failing to take risks, the ASWs were operating on a 'presumption of risk'; that is a belief that these situations were frequently unstable and inherently risky by virtue of the presence of the mental illness. Thus the ASWs did, albeit without great clarity, identify hazards placing patients at risk and their action, admitting the patient, indicated pessimism about likely future developments. These circumstances, *together with* the presence of mental illness, appear responsible for engendering a pessimistic outlook. Hence they often did not seem to analyse the cases in a way which would leave them more optimistic about the patient's prospects. An issue which connects both the lack of clarity and the 'presumption of risk' - the mental health orientation of the ASWs - will be discussed following further analysis.

It is evident that (a) the failure to separate hazard from danger and (b) the failure to identify the nature, degree and imminence of the danger contributes significantly to this process. Two factors, pessimism and lack of clarity in assessment, appear as integral elements of the 'presumption of risk'.

Type of Danger or Hazard and its Focus

The separation of danger from hazard is not sufficient in itself to indicate ASWs' interpretation of the health or safety of the patient or protection of others. Further analysis involves elucidation of the *nature* of the danger or hazard and *who* is its focus. Although involving different questions they are considered together, since it is clear from the ASWs' accounts that when indicating the danger or hazard they generally had to indicate *who* was at risk in order to render the account meaningful. Separation is therefore not only impractical in presenting these accounts but would misrepresent the ASWs' perceptions.

The various types of hazard or danger can be grouped broadly in terms of their focus: to the patient, to others and to patients and others.

To the Patient

a) *Patient Vulnerability* (19 cases) is a general term for the first type. This could take a number of forms. First, there were those *'out of control of themselves and their actions'*. A schizophrenic man had run around the neighbourhood naked and then hitched a lift to his sister's house (clothed). The lorry driver, quickly deciding he was mad, dropped him at the police station. The ASW said:

> 'He'd got himself into such a distressed and disturbed state that he was just running, not knowing what he was doing. He was wildly agitated with delusional ideas.'

Second, there were those open to *'exploitation by others'*. One schizophrenic woman was short of money. She was being harassed by men she knew who were demanding sex, and the ASW felt she may well provide it to get money, and that she was particularly vulnerable in this respect because of her illness. Likewise an eighteen year old suffering a manic episode:

> 'had been running around the village with no clothes on. She could have been raped or anything - it's full of marines in that area'.

Another man, a 'known manic depressive', was overactive and 'rushing around, practically without a break'. He was, the ASW said:

'spending money indiscriminately' and was 'very much at risk of being taken advantage of by unscrupulous people because of his immense generosity'.

Third, some laid themselves open to *'negative reaction'* from others. A manic woman, very active, not sleeping, and shouting and screaming and running about in the street, had 'verbally abused' her parents. The ASW commented:

> 'She was behaving irresponsibly.....it's very difficult for people to realise that someone behaving like that is sick, and they're likely to react in a negative way.'

This reaction is unclear, but presumably involved anything up to physical violence.

Finally, some patients suffered *'complete withdrawal'*. One woman had become depressed following a marital breakup and a positive cervical smear test. She had become increasingly withdrawn and found it difficult to cope with her three year old daughter. When seen by the ASW she had been:

> 'sitting in her car all morning. She was completely mute, holding tightly on to her daughter and her teddy bear. She was so distressed she just seemed to have cut herself off from everything'.

The vulnerabilities reflected the patient's relation to their environment, either in an inability to exercise some implicit level of control over their environment, or alternatively behaviour that might encourage responses by others with a deleterious effect.

b) Personal Neglect (5 cases) referred to a danger or hazard arising from omission rather than commission; the patient's standard of health and hygiene was as a result believed to place them at risk. One schizophrenic patient was considered to need treatment. The ASW commented - in relation to their health or safety - that:

> 'It's really the total neglect. He tends not to bother at all. His home is a tip, he hasn't got any idea about personal hygiene, he doesn't eat properly, and he's careless of where he goes and what he does'.

Another woman who was quite elderly believed her landlords were harbouring the IRA. The ASW was concerned, partly because of her age, that:

> 'she was beginning to neglect herself. She's got poor circulation and bad legs, so she can't afford to let herself go too much'.

The implication here is that age and physical infirmity reduces the threshold of risk, and that a section was necessary at an earlier stage than for a younger healthier person.

c) *Legal Risk* (2 cases). This relates to possible arrest and prosecution. One man, considered manic, was proclaiming that he would get the SAS to blow up a local landmark before the Queen's visit which, he thought, she would welcome. There was some suspicion that he had stolen maps from local stationers. The ASW said:

> 'I felt he was quite manic and that he was quite likely to get in trouble with the police with the way he was behaving.'

Another schizophrenic man was found in a local college looking into desks and taking various objects from them. He had no familial support and was referred by the police. The ASW felt that 'he was at risk of a burglary charge' if he was not hospitalised.

d) *Mental Health* (7 cases). This is an interesting interpretation of 'health or safety' which is nonetheless supported by the Mental Health Act Commission (1987). Thus they positively advocate detention when the patient's mental health deteriorates advising that this satisfies the criterion that detention should be for the patient's own health or safety. In order to be sectioned, the patient must already be suffering a mental disorder. If this is a mental illness (e.g. schizophrenia) this interpretation would allow the patient to be sectioned *simply because* they were mentally ill. The presence of extra criteria - that admission should be for the patient's health or safety - would appear to be superfluous.

The way this was interpreted, furthermore, varied with different cases. In some cases the *fear of deterioration* was primary. One man, living with his family, was no longer going to work although he was usually employed. The ASW commented that:

> 'His mental health state was deteriorating rapidly. He was paranoid and not taking medication.'

Likewise, an elderly woman was sectioned who:

> 'was known to have schizophrenic illness and stopped taking her medication. I felt she needed the medication to stop her getting worse'.

More vaguely, an ASW commented of a schizophrenic woman that:

> 'She's been refusing treatment, although she's been in hospital in the past. I felt she was a mental health risk'.

Alternatively, the patient was *already clearly mentally ill.* One woman was living alone but currently had psychiatric nursing support. The ASW said that:

> 'Her mental health was very poor. Judging from previous reports she was a together lady, quite able to manage her finances, home, life and so on'.

Another man was sectioned because:

> 'He was deluded with religious ideas. He said he had seen visions of the end of the world. He was totally out of touch with reality. He'd had a breakdown 30 years ago and had taken a long time to recover'.

The ASW added:

> 'I think anyone with a schizophrenic disorder is potentially a danger to themselves.'

A characteristic common to all these cases was that they had had a previous episode of mental illness. It may be, then, that a patient will generally be sectioned for a mental illness *alone* only in the presence of previous episodes. Furthermore, only psychotic patients were sectioned in this way, whereas in this and other studies a minority of the *total* group were sectioned for neurotic disorders.

Nonetheless, it raises an interesting issue. These admissions are clear examples of, in Bean's (1980) terminology, a 'treatment' orientation. All these patients were seen to be mentally ill, and it was their need for treatment which provided the rationale for admission. If so, this indicates an even greater accretion of power by ASWs and doctors than is implied by the additional criteria of the health or safety of the patient or protection of others, which appear to give protection against admission on the grounds of mental illness *alone* .

No doubt such admissions are only carried out in fairly serious circumstances - perhaps apparent by their psychotic state. However, once this principle is adopted there appears nothing to prevent compulsory admission of patients suffering *any* mental illness - whether psychotic or neurotic. These were people, it should be remembered, who, from the ASWs' accounts, represented no threat to others, nor to their own *physical* health or safety.

It appears some further guidelines are necessary. At present mutually contradictory positions appear to be adopted. For while clearly in some cases the ASW felt required to justify admission in terms of health or safety criteria *additional* to mental health, in other cases they did not. Either the criteria of health or safety of the patient or the protection of others is superfluous - and the logic of this is that they should be removed from the Act - or it is necessary to identify more clearly those circumstances where admission for mental illness *alone* is appropriate. In order to be open in this respect, this would become part of the Act, or at the very least published in a similar way to the guidelines provided in the DHSS (1983) *Memorandum,* as with, for example, the duty to interview 'in a suitable manner'. However, if this involves comments on the nature or severity of the mental illness this would appear to intrude on clinical judgement, which the Act appears reluctant to do.

Alternatively, mental illness *alone* may not be considered sufficient justification for compulsory admission. If so, the Act should require the presence of *physical* ill health or safety of the patient as the pertinent criteria. Of course, individual circumstances are sufficiently complex to require the exercise of sound judgement. But goodwill is not on its own sufficient, for the way this is exercised in different situations - for example, leaning towards the need for treatment or the preservation of liberty - will, as will become increasingly apparent from further analysis, depend on the orientation of the professionals involved. Whichever alternative is adopted, we are on the horns of a dilemma - but failure to be open about which 'rules' are being adopted leads to obfuscation rather than good judgement. This is unfair on the patients - the very people in whose interests the professionals consider themselves to be working.

It will be argued later (Part Four; Section 4) that this dilemma cannot, in fact, be resolved by reference to health alone. In order to make sense of the Mental Health Act Commission's position, a further concept - that of social functioning - must be introduced. This relates to role performance. This, it should be emphasised, is a *proposed* solution. However, it has significant implications, for it will require either further guidance on the interpretation of the legislation or amendment to the Act itself. All this will be discussed in more detail later.

To Other People (Protection of Others)

Certain kinds of situations fall *exclusively* into the 'protection of others' category. The most frequently identified group here (nine cases) was *'sub mental health distress or emotional trauma'*. In these cases, while there was no mention of others' mental health, the terminology used and the circumstances described indicated severe emotional pressure and the possibility of the person 'cracking up'. A good example was of the husband of a manic woman who was not sleeping, was emotionally labile, crying a great deal and absolutely convinced he was an alcoholic. She constantly accused him of drinking until he:

> 'felt he couldn't cope any more. He really was at breaking point'.

In addition to this she had lost weight and he was worried about this. The ASW said:

> 'He was quite desperate and didn't know what to do at all. She dominates him completely, so he was very distraught and tearful.'

Had the woman not been hospitalised the ASW did not know what her husband would do next.

These kind of terms appear consistently in these cases. Thus in one case the husband 'could no longer cope'. In another 'he was getting to the end of his tether', while another (wife) 'was getting really uptight about coping with him (the patient)'. Another woman:

> 'had been mentally worn down by him (the patient). She couldn't take any more. She said if he didn't go, she would'.

Throughout these cases the imagery of desperation in the carer pervades, caused largely by the behaviour of the patient.

The *'integrity of the family unit'* (two cases) is another category. One manic woman was up all night accusing her husband of hating her and plotting to get custody of the children. She was additionally muttering and making incongruous statements. The ASW said:

> 'Both the husband and the children were under a lot of pressure - there was a real danger she would break up the family. Her husband couldn't leave her at home with the children, but he couldn't stay off work for ever.'

In the circumstances he was likely to leave with the children, creating for her a self-fulfilling prophesy.

Another woman, also manic, was adamant that her husband was having an affair with his daughter-in-law. Both she and her husband were very distressed. She was constantly active and was not sleeping. The combination of this hyperactivity and the accusation had left 'the family unit at breaking point', thus she was admitted to hospital.

A final, interesting interpretation of protection of others relates to the *'reputation of a public figure'* (one case). A manic woman was making bizarre allegations in writing that a public figure was 'forcing children into prostitution'. She had in the past had a history of obsessive pursuit of a doctor and the ASW felt she might be tenacious in pursuit of the allegations. When sectioned she was about to make these allegations formally and in public, and she was admitted for this reason.

To the Patient and Others

Some dangers or hazards were common to both the patient and other people. There were numerous examples of possible *injury or death* (thirty cases). One man had become very aggressive and violent. The ASW cited in evidence that:

> 'He had dangerously scratched his wrists. He thought he was "dead hard" and both his hands were broken where he'd been banging on the walls'.

He had also banged his head on a police station cell wall. Another man, believing he would be reborn, had already cut his throat; while a woman, severely depressed, had slashed her wrists.

The risk to others was also evident: more frequently it was someone close to the patient - spouse, parent or children. One dramatic example was of a woman with pueperal psychosis, admitted informally, but who would have been sectioned had she refused, who screamed down the telephone:

> 'You must help me. I might kill my baby.'

The ASW commented that she was not sleeping, claiming her boyfriend was evil and 'getting at her', and had delusions that the baby was evil too. The admission was to protect the baby whom she had come close to killing by drowning in the bath.

Likewise, a morbidly jealous man was picked up by the police complaining of his wife's supposed misdemeanours. He was paranoid and 'everywhere he went he was shouting that his wife was a low bellied whore'. The ASW felt there was no option to sectioning because he was threatening to murder his wife and the man with whom she was supposed to be involved.

Possible death was not the only danger, however; in a number of cases it was physical injury. One man, becoming steadily more agitated, had attacked his wife twice and threatened her with a knife; another had punched his wife; while a manic woman was aggressive and 'violent to her (eighteen year old) daughter'.

Less frequently the danger was outside the family. Neighbours could be the target, as in the case of one man, increasingly manic and threatening, who had also thrown a broken bottle through his neighbours' window; or a woman, quite paranoid, who had hit an elderly neighbour the day before. Those professionally involved could also be the target. Thus one man had punched the electricity meter reader, while community psychiatric nurses were also attacked in other cases. The threat could be more broadly to a 'generalised other'. Thus one woman was considered 'very unpredictable'. She was:

> 'very hostile and threatening, throwing things at people, and had waved a kitchen knife at some people'.

Another psychotic woman had, in past psychotic episodes, taken a car

> 'and decided there were certain people who should be driven off the motorway'.

She promptly rammed six cars!

A second area is a broader one of *physical health* (23 cases). Here the *behaviour* of the person precipitated ill health, or the threat of it. One anorexic woman had been 'dieting' for some time, precipitated by a comment from her aunt that she was fat and ugly. The ASW said:

> 'She wasn't eating and had lost a lot of weight. She was pretty thin anyway, and there were signs of muscle wastage.'

A depressed woman had also stopped eating and drinking and there was a fear of kidney failure. The ASW commented:

> 'It was a problem of physical deterioration rather than killing herself',

Another schizophrenic woman, isolated and restless, 'appeared close to the point of exhaustion'.

The danger to other people's health generally possessed two characteristics: it focussed on the spouse, and they were *already vulnerable* through existing, and serious, ill health. One depressed woman, who was becoming increasingly agitated and crying said, 'You can't help me, I'll never get better'. She had a husband disabled with Parkinson's disease. The ASW felt:

> 'His physical health was threatened by Mrs. B's condition. Her behaviour caused a high level of stress, and there was no means of defusing it'.

With another hyperactive manic woman, the ASW felt:

> 'Her husband was at risk. He'd had a recent heart attack and I was really worried about the anxiety provoked by his wife'.

Likewise another man, who had angina, was finding it impossible to manage his verbally abusive, demented wife and was a physical risk.

In all these cases the behaviour of the spouse was considered stressful and, given the particular physical ill health, likely to act as a precipitator of relapse.

Focus for the Danger or Hazard

Overall it is helpful to indicate who was the focus for the danger or hazard. In the majority of cases it was the patients' health or safety. Additionally others may be grouped thus:

> The Spouse
> The Offspring (baby or child)
> The Family Unit
> Neighbours
> Officials or Professionals
> 'Generalised Others'
> Combination of more than one group

Comments Relating to Legal Interpretation

Clearly, from the ASWs' actions, a variety of possible circumstances relating to the health or safety of the patient or the protection of others may qualify patients for compulsory admission. Professor Hoggett has pointed to the lack of case law in this area which the ASW may use to guide their actions. Law texts, however, when addressing this area have taken either a *wider* or *narrower* interpretation of statute. In relation to 'health or safety of the patient' the main texts show little disagreement. Thus both Hoggett (1984) and Jones (1988) take a wide interpretation, while Anderson-Ford and Halsey (1984) do not comment in detail. Hoggett argues that because the Act does not use the term 'dangerous' to themselves - referring to possible death or injury - that a broad interpretation is appropriate: thus in relation to Section 3 ,once the doctor decides a patient needs treatment in hospital, it follows that this is necessary in the interests of his own health or safety.

Three different positions, however, are evident in relation to 'protection of others'. Anderson-Ford and Halsey take a narrow interpretation. They suggest this only refers to patients who, if discharged from hospital, would be likely to commit *acts of violence* to other persons. Hoggett, however, suggests the law allows psychiatrists a very wide interpretation - and this may include irritation and nuisance suffered by neighbours. The only confident statement that may be made, she suggests, is that 'the protection of property alone is not enough'. Jones takes a position between these two: that protection relates to both physical harm *and* emotional strain; thus irritation and nuisance suffered by neighbours is not sufficient.

When interpretations involving even such general statements vary so greatly, this serves to emphasise the looseness of the criteria of the Act. If we examine the admissions as a whole, they suggest that Hoggett's wide interpretation is adopted, at least by some ASWs. Thus, although a high proportion of cases involved possible ill health, injury or death, issues like the reputation of a public figure and family disruption were also included. Likewise in relation to 'health or safety' a wide variety of reasons are adopted. This does not, however, mean that *all* ASWs adopted a wide interpretation of the Act - indeed inconsistencies which will be discussed in the 'threshold of risk' section indicate that at times ASWs adopted a narrow interpretation of the Act.

Levels of Risk

All situations have some element of uncertainty, hence it is not possible to envisage a condition totally free from potential harm. It is necessarily the case, therefore, that the Act is concerned with the risk *over and above* some acceptable level in relation to the health or safety of the patient and the protection of other persons.

Risk assessment carries within itself two related elements: prediction and probability. Brearley's (1984) definition of risk as the 'relative variation in possible loss outcomes' indicates the elements of uncertainty. For our purposes it is useful to see risk as a link between hazard and danger: its level indicates the likelihood of the danger actually occurring in the face of the particular hazard. Hence the assessment of risk involves an element of prediction.

This is not, of course, an exact science. While the actuary may wish to calculate precisely the likelihood of particular outcomes in relation to certain populations, this is not available to ASWs. First, the ASW is not concerned with total populations but with particular individuals in situations which may appear complex. Second, we do not have precise figures for levels of risk in relation to particular dangers with which ASWs are concerned.

Hence it is not surprising the ASWs did not state the probability of the dangers occurring with any great precision. This is compounded by the fact that the ASW frequently identified a hazard rather than danger, making a reference point more difficult to distinguish. Thus the analysis of risk implicit in ASW actions involved broad qualitative distinctions indicating greater or lesser likelihood of undesired outcomes. These may be divided into four groups:

1. Demonstrated Danger

2. Probable or Latent Danger

3. Uncertain but Dangerous

4. Uncertain and Unclear

Demonstrated Danger **(21 cases)**

The first characteristic of this group is that the danger about which the ASW is concerned is already happening or has already happened. Some kind of damage may well have occurred. This means that the *current situation* rather than some future predicted possibility is that which is to be avoided. In addition to this, the ASW is implicitly expecting this to continue. A second characteristic arising from this is that compulsory admission occurs to stop some current form of behaviour, rather than prevent some possible future occurrence. Metaphorically, in terms of behaviour (as well as illness), the orientation is towards *cure* rather than prevention.

Thus, for example, a woman - psychotically depressed - believed a doctor was following her around in a car and preventing her seeing her children. She had attempted an overdose and said she did not wish to live. In other cases death was not the main concern: physical ill health or injury was already present. Thus one woman:

'wasn't caring for herself at all. She had no money, hadn't been eating for several days - she looked ill'.

Another hypomanic woman had left her husband:

'at breaking point.....he had hit her already that day and we were frightened he would injure her'.

In other cases patients were sectioned, as previously discussed, for already present mental illness. Although diverse, damage was already present in these cases - the overdose, injury and physical or mental ill health - and patients were sectioned to prevent their continuation or repetition.

Probable or Latent Danger (27 cases)

This group had four characteristics. Like the first group the danger concerning the ASW is clearly identified in their account. It does not require inference of the danger from the hazard. Second, but unlike the first group, there is no existing damage which the ASW hopes to discontinue. The damage has yet to occur - it is latent rather than actual, although given the circumstances it appears highly likely to occur. The circumstances point clearly in the direction of one particular danger to the exclusion of alternatives. That is, the situation described by the ASW is both consistent with the projected danger and makes it unlikely that alternatives will occur, whether they are alternative dangers or no danger at all. Finally, the emphasis of intervention is on prevention rather than cure: that is, to prevent some future outcome rather than to halt or discontinue some existing behaviour or damage.

One woman, severely depressed, had discontinued medication. She had become a recluse and believed she was being persecuted by neighbours who were sending messages through the walls. She had said that she did not want to live, and had made suicide attempts in past depressive episodes, although not during the current one. The ASW admitted her because she was 'actively suicidal'. This case shows the characteristics outlined. The danger (suicide) is clearly identified, it is latent rather than actual, the particular circumstances - depression, feeling of persecution, wishing to die and previous suicide attempts - all pointed to a particular danger and admission was to prevent the projected suicide (attempt).

Not all cases were that dramatic. One manic person who was not sleeping and had not stopped rushing about for days was admitted because:

> 'if she kept up at that rate she'd eventually collapse of fatigue'.

Another was:

> 'trying to pick fights with passers by and the chances are that somebody would have retaliated'.

Similarly another schizophrenic had not paid his rent for some time and was about to be made homeless through eviction. All, however, had the characteristics common to this group.

Uncertain but Dangerous (30 cases)

This group, like the latent danger group, was characterised by the fact that the danger had yet to occur. Thus like the last group it was necessary to surmise from existing circumstances the possibility of the danger actually occurring. However, unlike that group, a danger is not always clearly identified in the ASW's account; hence only the hazard may be identified. Because the danger was not clearly spelled out, there were occasions where its exact nature was unclear, although the fact that the person was potentially vulnerable to *some* kind of danger may be obvious. Third, the circumstances do not point clearly in the direction of a *particular* danger to the exclusion of alternatives. Instead, the danger is one of a number of alternative outcomes which may occur. This is emphasised most strongly where only the hazard is identified. Fourth, it is more difficult than with the 'latent danger' group to anticipate the likelihood of the danger occurring. The situation presented in the latent group made fairly clear that a particular danger was a likely outcome - everything appears to point in that direction. In the 'uncertain but dangerous' group, while possible dangers exist, the relationship between hazard and danger is not as clear cut - danger is one of a number of outcomes, the most likely of which is difficult to estimate. Finally, admission is to prevent some future danger rather than stop current damage.

One case demonstrates all these characteristics. An increasingly manic woman was not sleeping and described as 'very agitated'. She had become verbally abusive and had thrown various things out of the house, including books and food. The ASW commented that:

> 'She was in such a state she could have done anything. She really wasn't aware of what was going on around her. She could have crossed the road if she felt like it and would have been completely oblivious'.

Here the danger, a traffic accident, is implicit; it is one of a number of possible alternatives (might she have become exhausted, or hit someone throwing books?). Thus the danger is not clearly stated and there may be a number of alternative possibilities. The information does not indicate likelihood (has she walked in the main street recently? Did she dart into the road? Will she go out?). Finally, the danger has not yet occurred and admission is for prevention.

Other cases show similar characteristics: the demented octogenarian wandering off in the winter with 'no idea where he was'; the manic woman who, on past experience, was likely to drive her car, and whose driving, 'to put it mildly is rather erratic'; and a schizophrenic man:

> 'not so much physically violent to people, but throwing things about and making threatening gestures at them'.

Uncertain and Unclear (20 cases)

This group resembles the previous one in a number of respects: the danger - whatever it may be - has yet to occur; the emphasis in ASWs' accounts is on hazard rather than danger; and admission is to prevent future danger rather than stop current damage. However, a danger is never identified, although occasionally it is in the previous group. Second, the notion of the hazard makes it difficult to assess the degree of risk or indicates it is only possible. It is, therefore, a matter of degree; the danger appears less likely from the ASW account than in the previous group. In some cases an assumed danger may appear quite *unlikely* to occur.

One schizophrenic woman was overactive, shouting and constantly pacing up and down. She lived with her two children but had not threatened them. Her husband had felt the need to stay at home to look after the children. The ASW sectioned the woman because:

> 'She obviously needed help. There was nothing *specific* which threatened her - she wasn't suicidal or anything. I could imagine her wandering off and getting into predicaments though'.

This lack of specificity leaves us unsure of the degree of risk, and indeed what the danger was. Certainly if the ASW had justified admission on the grounds of *mental* health risk (as discussed earlier) a danger - schizophrenia - would have been identified. However, the ASW did not. Indeed the account dismisses other possible grounds, such as violence or suicidal feelings. Admission was justified by her 'wandering off and getting into predicaments'. However, *imagination* rather than evidence was the basis for this. Furthermore, if she had wandered off there is no evidence of *what* precisely these possible predicaments would be.

Overall, then, the account indicates a woman who is mentally ill, whose behaviour has disrupted the family but where it is very difficult to gauge the level of risk - if any - which she presents. Another example - of a schizophrenic woman quarrelling with her family - illustrates this

55

vagueness and emphasis on hazard. The ASW commented, in relation to the risk:

> 'It's difficult to say. She was causing problems with her neighbours and beginning to neglect herself a bit. The child (her nephew) could possibly have been at risk, but there was no evidence yet.'

In all these cases the vagueness of the account makes it difficult to assess the level of risk, or to indicate more than a small risk. It may be that the presentation of mental illness - all these patients were considered psychotic - was disturbing enough for the ASW, without adopting an exclusively treatment model not to consider clearly the nature of the danger or level of risk. If so this emphasises the difficult of assessment in crises, and that 'non-routine' situation may 'throw' the ASW no matter how frequently they are confronted. This further emphasises the 'presumption of risk' discussed previously.

Evidence

To a considerable extent the clarity with which hazards or dangers were identified was related to the evidence presented. The overwhelming majority of cases were characterised by evidence gained broadly from *information and observation* (83 cases); that is, evidence based on the patient's information about their beliefs, feelings or behaviour, or from others with a knowledge of the patient and their behaviour. Alternatively the evidence was based on direct observation of the patient by the ASW.

Some care should be taken with interpretation, for in asking the ASWs to provide their reasons for compulsory admission the question may imply the need for the collection of evidence based on awareness of the patient's current situation. Although the question was not of a 'why did you section them?' type they may nonetheless have sought justification for admission on this basis. However, on most occasions there was little hesitation, or only a brief pause for thought, by the ASW before replying, suggesting they had already considered their reasons. This contrasts with some cases identified by Bean (1980) where both social workers and GPs gave little thought to the section.

This group is of two types: in the first, the nature of the health or safety of the patient or protection of others was closely connected to, or part of, the mental illness itself. What is occurring here is that the social problems, although identified, are also being reinterpreted not as social problems but as indications of the presence of mental illness. They are, in a sense, the symptoms of the mental illness (cf. Bean, 1980). This is of some significance for the evidence serves two purposes: it provides evidence for the presence of mental illness *and* it provides grounds for perceiving a health or safety of the patient or protection of others threat.

This is apparent in the case of a manic man. He had run around the street at 2 a.m. banging on doors and windows. He had not been sleeping, had lost a great deal of weight since last seen by the ASW and believed 'the Russians were running the world from a biscuit tin'. He was sectioned because he was:

> 'so hyperactive that he wasn't eating or drinking - he wouldn't stop to do it. Or it wasn't that he wouldn't, it was just that he'd take one sip and be off'.

The danger was 'to his physical condition'. The hyperactivity, the failure to drink and eat, were seen both as symptoms of his manic state and as the threat to his health or safety.

Other cases showed a similar connection: as with the depressed woman, introverted and:

> 'not talking much. She wasn't contributing to home management. She wasn't eating or sleeping and said she wished she was dead'.

Or the schizophrenic woman with:

> 'paranoid delusions.....that she was being followed, a camera in her TV was watching her and the house was bugged'.

As a result she refused to return home - with nowhere else to go - and was becoming hostile to her husband when he suggested these beliefs were inaccurate.

In some cases, as previously discussed, mental ill health *was* the 'health or safety' threat justifying admission. This, then, represents a second way in which the distinction of mental disorders from 'health or safety' criteria is clouded. It is, however, more subtle for it appears they are separate while the evidence in fact serves a dual purpose.

This is not to suggest that these admissions were somehow 'wrong', but rather that the 'knowledge orientation' is significant for giving evidence meaning (Huntington, 1981). It emphasises the explanation of particular behaviour in medical terms, and indicates that such explanations have implications in terms of response. Had the evidence been interpreted differently - without recourse to psychiatry - the responses may have been different. Taken in conjunction with other areas - the 'uncertain and unclear' risk group, and mental illness as the 'health or safety' danger group - these ASWs, far from being anti-psychiatric as suggested by psychiatrists in Bean's study, positively embraced a psychiatric orientation.

The other form of information and observation was where evidence was not *directly* connected in this way with the mental illness, i.e. it did not serve the aforementioned dual purpose. In all these cases, the 'protection of others' was the focus. Some of the best examples have already been mentioned: as with the man who, because of his manic wife's behaviour was:

> 'quite desperate and didn't know what to do at all.....he
> was very distraught and tearful'.

Or the husband of a depressed woman who was 'at the end of his tether', or the case of the manic woman where:

> 'there was a real danger she would break up the family'
> because both 'the husband and the children were under
> a lot of pressure'.

These were considerably fewer in number - five - than the first type.

The second major area of evidence was based on *knowledge of the psychiatric condition* (seven cases). In these cases the ASW consciously connected the mental illness with the patient's behaviour, and used it as evidence. This reverses the relationship between mental illness and behaviour just discussed, where the evidence, in the form of behaviour, was used to indicate psychiatric symptoms. In this area, the behaviour was seen, so to speak, to follow on from the illness state. Thus the illness indicates the behavioural danger rather than the behaviour indicating the illness.

Thus, of one man in his late sixties, with whom his wife was finding it increasingly difficult to cope, the ASW said:

> 'He was running off in a demented state - he didn't know
> where he was. He had been found wandering and had
> been violent when his wife had tried to stop him. Really

he was a classic dementia. I think the only thing we could do was to get him into hospital. No one else could cope.'

In another case the link between depression and suicide was made:

'I did feel there was an underlying depressive illness. There was little to keep him carrying on, and he might have done himself in.'

Another woman:

'was really too high. In her state you couldn't rely on her staying in one place. She was like a lot of manics - overactive and likely to get aggressive'.

This explicit inference from mental state to future danger was not, however, frequent.

Finally, evidence based on *previous knowledge of the patient* was used: where explicit reference was made to behaviour during past episodes of mental illness to justify current admission. Of one manic woman, the ASW commented that she was likely to become disinhibited:

'In the past she had been at risk going out late and chatting up men. It hasn't happened so far, but on past performance I expect it would.'

In another case, of a depressed woman, the ASW commented that she 'is at high risk of suicide when in this state' and 'had made attempts in the past'; while in a further case, previously mentioned, the ASW referred to a past schizophrenic episode when the patient had tried to drive some people off the motorway and rammed six vehicles.

There were only seven of these cases and it is notable that 'previous knowledge' was never used on its own to justify admission, but as part of a collection of evidence.

THE THRESHOLD OF RISK: INCONSISTENCIES IN ASSESSMENT AND OUTCOME

The process of assessment for compulsory admission is clearly very complex. Fine distinctions are often made, and confusion between relevant areas - for example hazards and dangers - may deleteriously affect judgement. This serves to emphasise the need for conceptual clarity in the assessment process. Such clarity is essential when attempting to define an appropriate threshold, above which a patient is sectioned, and below which they are not. This appears to be a function of two things:

1. The seriousness of the danger.

2. The level of risk.

In relation to danger the problem may be serious, for example a suicide attempt, or less serious, spraining an ankle. The ASW may be little concerned by the latter, but very worried about the former. The ASW should be considerably more concerned about a possible suicide where there is a high risk of it occurring than when the risk is lower. This can be presented diagramatically:

	Serious Danger	Minimal Danger
High Risk	A	C
Low Risk	B	D

Box A represents serious danger - high risk, which might, for example, involve possible death or serious injury where the evidence is strong that the danger will actually occur. Box B, on the other hand, would involve a similarly serious danger, but where the ASW felt it was very unlikely to take place. Box C involves a minimal danger, which could be something which presented a mild health risk - perhaps a cold - of which there is a high risk, maybe because the person is wandering around in damp weather. Finally, Box D involves a similarly minimal danger where there is a low risk of even that kind of danger taking place. Clearly those in group A - if mentally ill and refusing admission - would be sectioned, or this would be the expectation created by the Act, as might *possibly* be the case with Group B. Those in Group D, and probably Group C, would not.

However, presenting risk and danger in this way simplifies the situation. We have, so far, only two sets of simple dichotomies: high and low risk, serious and minimal danger. In fact, for each of these factors there are 'grey areas' or gradations in which seriousness of danger and level of risk may be greater or lesser. When the two are related to each other the situation is endowed with much greater complexity. Both danger and risk are better presented as part of a spectrum (Figure 1).

Figure 1: Dimensions of Risk and Danger

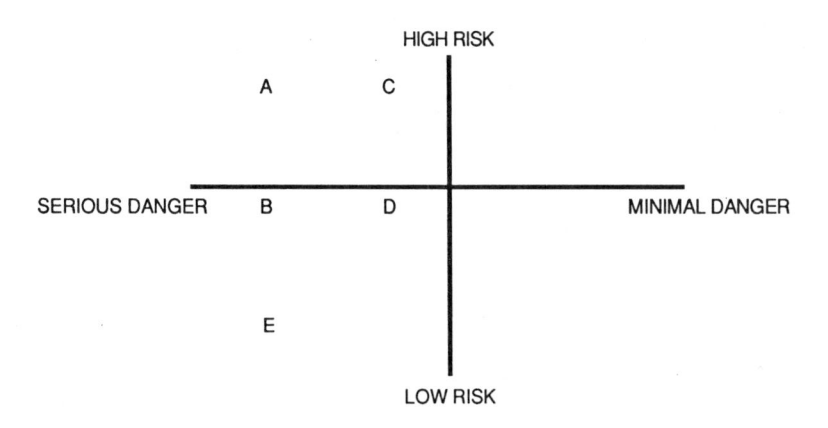

```
                          HIGH RISK
             A       C        |
                              |
   ─────────────────────────┼─────────────────────────
   SERIOUS DANGER  B    D    |         MINIMAL DANGER
                              |
                              |
                     E        |
                              |
                          LOW RISK
```

This diagram shows the greater complexity of the relationship between risk and dangers. Where the patient is in position A the situation is quite unproblematic: they are at high risk of serious danger. Positions B, C, D and E are more problematic: does the ASW section where they are at moderate risk of serious danger (position B)? What if they are at low risk of serious danger (position E), or at moderate risk of moderate danger (position D)? What if they are at high risk of moderate danger (position C)? Clearly, fine judgement is required by the ASW when deciding the threshold to admit.

Of course, this is presented abstractly, without identifying cases considered at high or low risk, or serious or minimal danger. However, it does highlight the 'grey' areas sometimes confronted, and reaffirms Davies' (1985) perception of social workers as 'brokers in shades of grey'. Difficult though this area is, it is of the greatest importance to the patient, for this concerns their civil rights. What if the likelihood of compulsory admission depends on which ASW is assessing? Or worse, what if individual ASWs varied in their judgement from day to day?

Both these in fact occurred. Altogether eleven patients were not sectioned under circumstances very similar to others who were. The nature of these cases, however, suggests the ASWs were not operating, at times, around a relatively narrow 'threshold' area but that inconsistencies could occur which included apparently serious danger and possibly high levels of risk. It is instructive to compare these with earlier examples with considerably less serious danger and more moderate risk.

In two cases individuals were not sectioned where, in the face of a mental disorder, a serious threat of injury to others was recognised. One man, whose behaviour was described by the ASW as 'very aggressive, even menacing' threatened them with a 'six shooter' under his coat.

The ASW, believing this, left and called the police, who would only come if a direct complaint was made which the ASW would not do. The ASW said:

> 'Perhaps in retrospect I could have sectioned him, but the violence may have clouded the issue.'

Another case was of a schizophrenic man with a past history of violence when he was ill, and the ASW was 'very, very wary of a likely explosion'. His neighbours had reported him to be banging on his wall and shouting. With only one approved doctor involved they decided not to admit him, although:

> 'We would have sectioned him if there had been a second doctor'.

They wanted police support which was not arranged and in its absence 'decided discretion was the better part of valour'. Apart from professional issues, like the duty to interview in a suitable manner, to section when appropriate and the allowable time lapse between medical recommendations, these were clearly criteria, possible injury or death, which in other circumstances led to admission. Furthermore, the types of evidence - current observation and information and previous knowledge of the patient - had been used elsewhere to admit patients compulsorily. Clearly, these were frightening situations, but there was a failure to make use of possible police protection. Indeed, in the first case the ASW apparently did not communicate to the police that such protection was to be part of a section assessment.

Other cases fitted into the 'patient vulnerability - exploitation by others' category. One schizophrenic woman was 'standing in the street showing her breasts to passers by' while another had 'been deteriorating for a while (and) had been out in the street approaching passers by suggesting they should go to bed with her'. The ASW here disagreed with the doctors who 'felt she might be raped any minute'.

Others fitted into the 'mental illness' danger category. One woman, floridly schizophrenic, was considered 'clearly mentally ill'. She was:

'picked up wandering the streets.....she said she thought her son had come into the bedroom to kill her, that blood was oozing out of the walls, and talked of a non-existent boyfriend'.

Additionally she 'looked very ill'. The ASW did not admit in this case despite the willingness of doctors and the additional possible illness.

Some of these cases do perhaps occupy a 'grey area' consistent with a relatively narrow 'threshold of risk'. This *might* be argued of the woman showing her breasts to passers-by although even this may be questionable. This would be more difficult to argue in relation to 'menacing' men, with possible dangers of injury or death. Nonetheless, these cases do indicate the pitfalls of entering an arena where values are so centrally involved without the necessary conceptual categories, and where the criteria for stepping over the 'threshold of risk' are not so much vague as non-existent. Social work in this area involves not just sound judgement, but needs also to be cerebral.

Overall, we can broadly divide the decision-making process into four. There is some overlap between these categories because the factors influencing the decisions were in some respects common. Hence, for example, there is a relationship between 'inconsistent' and 'uncertain' decisions, based on a lack of clarity of analysis.

Unproblematic decisions: where there were clearly stated dangers, or the way the hazards were stated made the danger quite obvious.

Inconsistent decisions: where patients were admitted in circumstances where others were not, reflecting a failure to apply the same standards to different cases, and a lack of clarity of analysis.

Maverick decisions: these were a particularly serious type of inconsistent decisions, where patients were not admitted in circumstances which the Act clearly intended to cover, and the consequences of failing to admit could have been very grave. This is most obvious in the two cases mentioned in the 'threshold of risk' section, where mentally disordered individuals were not sectioned where serious threat of injury to others was recognised. These cases raise serious questions about professional conduct.

Uncertain decisions: where the ASW accounts are quite unclear as to the nature or severity of the danger, or the level of risk to the patient.

Mentally Ill Patients Not Admitted

In addition to the patients not sectioned in circumstances very similar to others who were, there were a further six patients defined as mentally ill but not admitted. Three of these were considered schizophrenic, one depressed, one alcoholic, and one suffering an anxiety state. Admissions were refused on various grounds. The patients with alcohol problems did not come under the auspices of the Act (see Section 1), and the patient suffering anxiety was not considered mentally disordered (although it is defined as such in the World Health Organisation, *International Classification of Diseases*). In one case the patient, not previously known to the psychiatric services, was only provisionally diagnosed as schizophrenic, and there remained some uncertainty.

> 'She was acting strangely and our provisional diagnosis was schizophrenia. But it was very mild and the GP could monitor her and call for a section assessment if necessary'.

In all other cases (two schizophrenic and one depressed) the patient was previously known to the psychiatric services. The two schizophrenic patients were considered schizophrenic because of a previous diagnosis on the assumption that 'once a schizophrenic always a schizophrenic' but they were not symptomatic when interviewed. Hence the label attached to these patients owed less to their current behaviour than to assumptions about the nature of schizophrenia. Being asymptomatic they could as easily not have been considered schizophrenic. Thus, the patient in one case was:

> 'not sufficiently mentally ill at that stage. He was probably not delusional, although he was very disruptive and shouting'.

The other patient was:

> 'a well known schizophrenic but is not symptomatic at the moment'.

Both, furthermore, agreed to take medication. In the final case of a depressed woman, she had also agreed to take medication and was not seen as an immediate threat to herself or others.

Disagreements between ASWs and Doctors

The ASWs clearly - as a group - adopted a wide variety of interpretations of the 'health or safety of the patient' and the 'protection of other persons', while at the same time showing some inconsistency in applying the law. However, these decisions were not made in isolation from the medical assessments. Current theory relating occupational culture to social work and medical practice suggests there is considerable scope for disagreement between ASWs and doctors (Pavalko, 1971; Huntington, 1981; Bean, 1980). Did such disagreement occur with compulsory admission assessment? A second issue relating to this is the question of whether or not the doctors were themselves more consistent in their application of the law.

The concentration of the research on the ASWs' accounts does not allow direct access to the doctors' view of what took place. However, the ASWs were asked if disagreement occurred between the professionals, and if so what were the alternative positions adopted?

In terms of all 120 patients, whether admitted compulsorily or informally or not at all, there were only 10 cases where disagreement occurred. This in itself indicates a remarkable concurrence which is emphasised still further when it is recognised that the majority of assessments involved two doctors as well as the ASW, and that all but one of the compulsory admissions required two doctors, since they involved Sections 2 and 3 of the Act. This level of agreement indicated by the ASWs suggested that the doctors involved adopted very similar perspectives to those of the ASWs. This is perhaps not surprising because a considerable number of cases display a 'mental health orientation' amongst the ASWs. The nature of the mental health orientation and the basis for suggesting ASWs adopted such an orientation will be discussed in more detail later. However, it involves placing a greater emphasis on the patient's mental health status than the issue of the 'health or safety of the patient' or 'protection of other persons'. Such an emphasis on the health and treatment needs of the patient would appear natural for the medical practitioner, and fits with current knowledge about medicine.

The ASWs, therefore, in many cases - although not always - adopted an orientation characteristic of medicine. This may contribute to the explanation of the inconsistencies and wide interpretation of the criteria of the 'health or safety of the patient' and 'protection of others' by the ASWs. The high level of agreement between ASWs and doctors suggests the latter also interpreted these criteria widely and that they also showed some inconsistency in the decisions they made.

The disagreements that did occur were of four types:

1. About whether or not to section the patient (6 cases).
2. About whether or not the patient was mentally ill (1 case).
3. About whether to admit informally or compulsorily (2 cases).
4. About which section on which to admit the patient compulsorily (1 case).

Most were not acrimonious disagreements. In one case neither the ASW nor the psychiatrist felt the patient was sectionable, but while the ASW felt she was 'quite eccentric and that people should be allowed to behave as they wish', the psychiatrist considered her to be 'a woman who has been schizophrenic, but was no longer taking Modecate and was showing signs of mental illness and would eventually deteriorate'.

On another occasion, when both the psychiatrist and the ASW agreed the patient was depressed and should be admitted to hospital, the psychiatrist wanted her admitted under Section 2. However, following a lengthy interview the ASW 'discovered she would go in informally and argued for this'. The psychiatrist reluctantly agreed because the ASW would not fill in the application under these circumstances. In a further case, both doctors and the ASW agreed the patient should not be sectioned, but while the ASW felt she should be admitted, the psychiatrist did not. The ASW thought there 'might be things below the surface which she had not admitted', and that further assessment would be helpful.

However, in some cases the ASW was more critical. One psychiatrist referred a man who was in general hospital and was 'a living skeleton'. He had undergone major surgery and was not responding, and was considered depressed. The ASW considered this 'the worst referral I'd ever had'. The referral had come secondhand through the psychiatrist's secretary, and the psychiatrist had already visited and signed the medical recommendation for a section without consulting the ASW, presenting her with a *fait accompli*. What marked it out, however, was that:

'The man was distressed and dying.....he was so weak, so feeble and ill. He was scared and had been crying'.

He was being visited by relatives when the ASW appeared. The psychiatrist wanted admission so that he could be given Electro

Convulsive Therapy (ECT) for depression which the ASW considered 'totally inappropriate'.

On another occasion a GP referred a man who had recently undergone major surgery, and relatives had contacted him 'looking for something to cope with the side effects of medication'. The GP, who did not visit the patient, was considered 'incompetent' by both the ASW and the psychiatrist who visited. They did not admit the patient, who showed no signs of mental disorder, and they felt the referral by the GP was to 'get them (the relatives) off his back'. Another case was viewed similarly. The GP, who had made the referral, wanted a woman who was depressed to be admitted compulsorily. However, both ASW and psychiatrist did not consider her a risk to herself or to others, and when offered voluntary admission she refused. The ASW felt, as with the previous example, the referral was really 'to get her off his (the GP's) back'.

All these cases show that in some circumstances the ASW was prepared to take independent decisions. The exercise of this independence, especially in relation to a psychiatrist, could be a source of pride. In one case a consultant wanted compulsory admission, even though the patient had agreed to informal admission. When pressed to sign, the ASW said:

'I wouldn't, and I didn't, and I feel quite smug about that!'

However, differences were rare, and on the few occasions where they were serious the ASW's account suggests serious professional incompetence by the doctor. Furthermore, as the examples show, division frequently did not occur along occupational lines: the ASW would agree with one doctor but not the other. On the whole, therefore, the degree of agreement suggests that the assessments were characterised by shared perspectives between the ASWs and doctors.

Comment

The apparently straightforward criteria of 'health or safety of the patient' and 'protection of other people' are clearly, in their practical application, a matter of great complexity. It is not a simple matter of applying 'objective' and easily understandable principles which patients can be sure will be applied with reasonable uniformity. Rather it is a matter of the construction placed on it by the ASWs.

It is, first of all, value laden. The fact that there may be considerable agreement about many of these values should not obscure this. This need not be a problem for social work. Indeed, I have argued elsewhere that social workers are, because of the nature of their work, always necessarily committed to value positions (Sheppard, 1982). They cannot opt out of this commitment. However, their task is to be clear about these values, and to be able to justify them. Thus, preventing death may present few value dilemmas, whereas the 'integrity of the family' is rather more on the margins as an excuse for deprivation of liberty. Certainly many families *without* mentally ill members separate in acrimonious circumstances without any member being deprived of their liberty (by, for example, imprisonment).

However, these values are not always consistently applied. This relates both to those areas which may legitimately be regarded as representations of the 'health or safety of the patient' or 'the protection of other persons' *and* to the degree of seriousness of those problems. This was evident where some patients were sectioned in circumstances where others were not. Furthermore, even in situations where inconsistencies were not identified, some sections may be more difficult to justify than others - particularly where there was no obvious danger.

The ASWs also, in a number of ways, demonstrated a 'mental health' orientation. The essence of the mental health orientation is a considerably greater emphasis on the mental health or disorder of the patient than on the issue of the health or safety of the patient or protection of other persons, to the detriment of the latter. This does not mean that the health or safety of the patient or protection of others were disregarded, but that the mental health state was given greater importance in the judgement about compulsory admission. This is not obvious in the relatively clear-cut cases, where dangers were serious and stated, or at least obvious, based on the ASWs description of the hazard. These cases were relatively unproblematic. It is clearest in the 'uncertain and unclear' group, i.e. where decisions were more problematic, where although a mental disorder was present the health or safety of the patient or protection of others danger was far from obvious. This was furthermore positively embraced in a variety of other ways: patients were sectioned simply for being mentally ill. The behaviour of patients indicating a health or safety of the patient or protection of others danger was also used to indicate the presence of mental illness (the evidence serving a dual purpose), and knowledge of mental illness was used to infer likely future dangers.

This 'mental health orientation' which is itself a value position helps explain the therapeutic orientation adopted in many cases by the ASWs. The presence of the mental illness appeared for the ASW to transform situations which in other circumstances may not have been considered risky into potentially risky situations. This 'presumption of risk', then, appears closely related to the perceived presence of mental illness. Where people were being sectioned, where the danger was unclear (and in twenty of the relevant cases this occurred), this effectively meant that the ASWs' primary concern was to obtain treatment for the patient. The presumption in many of these cases was that such treatment would reduce the risk to the health or safety of the patient or protection of others. The ASWs' approach in many cases is similar to that of psychiatrists, described by Bean (1980), and would be expected to reduce considerably the likelihood of conflict between the two professions. Certainly the image of the ASW as suspicious of mental health labels and 'over concerned' about patients' civil rights is not borne out by this research. Furthermore, although when conducting these assessments the ASWs were working from the Mental Health Advice Centre, a number of them were based in area teams and worked at the Centre from time to time on the basis of a rota. It would be a mistake, therefore, to assume that area team social workers would approach matters differently simply because they were not based in a Mental Health Advice Centre. Indeed, the ASW training may have developed an understanding and sympathy for mental health issues amongst social workers not apparent before the 1983 Act.

The research raises important policy issues. Insofar as the 1983 Act, like the 1959 Act, is concerned with *mental health,* the ASWs' orientation will be welcomed. However, specific problems arise in relation to the interpretation of 'health or safety of the patient' where it includes mental health. Certainly, the situation advocated by the Mental Health Act Commission, and adopted in some cases by these ASWs, leads to inconsistencies and suggests further guidelines are badly needed. More generally, the inconsistencies apparent in some of the ASWs' decisions, as well as their vagueness with a considerable minority of the patients in identifying the nature of the danger, suggests the process of assessment, in terms of the social circumstances at least, would benefit from greater rigour. Furthermore, the ASWs rarely found themselves in disagreement with the doctors. It is worth noting that most of these cases involved detailed discussions with doctors, and that where lack of clarity was present this may well have been reflected in the doctors' thinking.

Furthermore, the complexity of these assessments has implications for the nearest relative's position as applicant. Their position is in many respects already anomalous in view of the training required by ASWs. The fact that the ASWs at times struggled with very difficult judgements makes the position of the nearest relative still more questionable. It is perhaps time to recognise that the nearest relative is not really equipped to make these assessments. This issue will be considered in more detail later.

'Mental Health' Versus 'Social Risk' Orientations

One possible conclusion from the research is that at least two distinct orientations are possible which will be called a 'mental health orientation' and a 'social risk' orientation. Although related to Bean's 'treatment' and 'legal' models, they are different. First, they refer only to the interpretation of health or safety of the patient or protection of others, and second they refer to the relative weight attached to 'mental disorders' versus 'health or safety of the patient or protection of others'. It is not a matter of whether legal rules are followed or broken or whether there is recourse to courts, since it is already clear - even from legal commentators - that wide interpretations of the health or safety of the patient or protection of others is possible. Thus, it is not a matter of breaking the spirit or letter of the law; rather one of emphasis *within* the law.

Anderson-Ford and Halsey (1984) suggest both that the 1983 Act was more civil liberation than its predecessor, and that the clearer ASW role is intended to balance the power of the medical profession. However, to achieve these aims, two elements are required:

1. ASWs should develop a social risk orientation, rather than a mental health orientation.

2. They should develop an appropriate conceptual framework to analyse risk.

These two orientations are summarised in Figure 2. It should be emphasised they are ideal types and are best perceived as tendencies which may be manifested to a greater or lesser extent in assessments.

Mental Health Orientation

1. Places greater emphasis on mental health status; gives health/safety/protection of others subordinate status.

2. health/safety/protection of others frequently seen as an aspect of mental illness itself. In particular:

a) including mental illness as an aspect of health or safety;

b) close interchange-ability between mental illness and its perceived health/safety/ protection of others implications (dual purpose of evidence)

3. Reduces perceived need for clear analysis of health/safety/protection of others. Less clarity both in analysis and decision-making on health/safety/protection of others grounds.

4. Tends towards pessimistic outlook for patients.

5. An increased likelihood of a 'presumption of risk' occurs, particularly where health/safety/protection of others analysis is unclear.

6. Tends towards a wide 'threshold of risk' because of unclear analysis (at times).

7. Possible 'admission by default'.

Social Risk Orientation

1. Gives the assessment of health/safety/protection of others equal status to mental health.

2. Emphasises the need to examine health/safety/ protection of others independently and in its own right.

3. Affirms need for clear identification of precisely what dangers, hazards and risks are involved.

4. Neither pessimistic nor optimistic - emphasis on realistic.

5. No preconceptions exist about risk - emphasises conclusions based on evidence.

6. A narrower 'threshold of risk' is likely because of clearer assessment.

7. No admission without clear evidence.

The social risk orientation emphasises strongly the clear and careful assessment of factors related to the health or safety of the patient or protection of others. It is called 'social risk' because these factors invariably involve the behaviour of the individual in their social context and/or their interrelations with others. Dangers and risks are generally created by acts of omission or commission on the part of the individual. Furthermore, they are assessed, as we have seen in Part One, within a framework of what is socially defined as problematic (social problems).

The social risk orientation is most definitely *not* anti-psychiatric, where this involves the wholesale denial of the validity of the concept of mental illness. It does not, furthermore, preclude recognition of the health or safety of the patient or protection of others implications of mental disorders. However, it does emphasise the need to assess health or safety of the patient or protection of others rigorously and in its own right. This involves two elements: having the conceptual tools to do it and perceiving section assessment as a two stage process in which diagnosis of mental disorder is followed by (metaphorically) 'diagnosis' of the 'health or safety of the patient' or 'protection of other persons'.

To some extent this involves a division of labour. Although the ASW should have some understanding of mental disorder, and is involved in its assessment, the primary role will normally be that of the Approved Doctor (although both research (Bean, 1980) and experience indicate some GPs may be less competent than ASWs in assessing mental disorders). However, the ASW would be expected, through the development of an appropriate conceptual framework, to take the lead in assessing risk. Why is this?

Quite simply because mental health and social risk orientations are to a considerable degree mutually exclusive. We would expect that doctors - simply because of their training (Huntington, 1981) - would on the whole veer towards a mental health orientation. Indeed, research on the 1959 Act shows some psychiatrists operated therapeutic rules which emphasised the need for treatment (Bean, 1980). This is closely related to the mental health orientation outlined here.

Social workers, however, appear well qualified to take on this role. First, they are involved in the assessment of serious risk in various aspects of their work - including child care and the elderly, as well as mental health. Second, risk is conceptualised as part of a social process, with social causes, progress and effects, which is quite clearly separate from a 'biophysical' orientation (Huntington, 1981). Third, risk analysis is not reliant on a medical foundation alone; it owes its allegiance also to a psychosocial foundation and is, therefore, in part at least *independent* of medicine. This is dependent, in the last analysis, on the independent knowledge base of social work; placed as it is on the foundation of social science knowledge (Sheppard, 1984).

The ASW assessment, potentially at least, is one truly independent of the medical assessment. This could not, for example, be said of the psychiatric nurse, even with the new community training. They tend - perhaps inevitably because of the chronology and emphasis of their training - to emphasise a 'medical model' and show far less ability to analyse and act on complex social situations than social workers (Woof, 1987). Their training leaves them in a subordinate position to the dominant medical profession, which defines their area of work, and leaves them with an orientation similar to that of psychiatrists. For social workers, as ASWs, on the other hand, the assessment of risk in a mental health situation is only one aspect of the assessment of risk in a variety of situations, and is founded on an independent knowledge base which owes its strength to the understanding and flexible use of the social sciences (Sheppard, 1984).

As a final point, this provides an example of the first rank importance of a social science knowledge base to social work. Without a strong allegiance to, and an understanding of, this area the ASW is likely to be overwhelmed by the powerful 'medical model' when assessing for compulsory admission. In this area, therefore, we have provided strong indications that Davies (1985) is wrong to perceive social science knowledge as marginal to social work.

The second element necessarily related to the social risk orientation is the importance of clarity in making assessments. This of course has implications for ASW training. While only some cases suffered from lack of clarity, they were sufficient to be of concern. The framework adopted here, using risk analysis, may provide the basis for improvement. Although further refinements are necessary to develop useful knowledge in this area, it is helpful at this stage provisionally to summarise the main areas which have been identified here, in the form of a typology of the ways in which the health or safety of the patient or protection of others is interpreted in practice.

1. DANGERS AND HAZARDS:

a) Danger clearly indicated
b) Hazard indicated/Danger obvious
c) Hazard indicated/Danger unclear

2. TYPES OF DANGER AND HAZARD:

To patient:

a) Patient vulnerability
b) Personal neglect
c) Legal risk
d) Mental health

To other people:

a) Sub mental health distress/emotional trauma
b) Integrity of family unit
c) Reputation of a public figure

To patient & others

a) Injury or death
b) Physical health

3. FOCUS FOR DANGER OR HAZARD:

a) Patient
b) Offspring (baby or child)
c) Family unit
d) Neighbours
e) Officials/professionals
f) 'Generalised others'

4. LEVELS OF RISK:

a) Demonstrated danger
b) Probable/latent danger
c) Uncertain but dangerous
d) Uncertain and unclear

5. EVIDENCE:

a) Information/observation
b) Knowledge of psychiatric condition
c) Previous knowledge of patient

This typology provides a guide to the way that ASWs *actually behaved* and hence makes manifest the various ways they used the criteria of 'health or safety of the patient' and 'protection of other persons'. However, this takes us only so far because, as with dangers and hazards, the typology inevitably reflects the lack of clarity evident in some of their work, and also because it is helpful to go further than a simple typology if we are to develop a more sophisticated and flexible way of assessing in practice the 'health or safety of the patient' and 'protection of other persons'. This is the task which will be taken up in the next part.

PART THREE

A SCHEDULE FOR ASSESSING COMPULSORY ADMISSIONS

The research so far has demonstrated the importance of clarity of analysis when assessing for compulsory admission, and that frequently this clarity of analysis is missing. When this occurs there is a danger of 'admission by default' where, although undertaken entirely in good faith, admission occurs without any clear idea of danger.

This possibility is made more likely by the unequal relationship between the criteria for assessing mental disorder and that for assessing the 'health or safety of the patient' or 'protection of others'. The lack of 'knowledge' guidelines for assessing the health or safety of the patient or protection of others stands in stark contrast to the carefully developed symptomatology for assessing mental disorder. This appears to contribute significantly to the mental health orientation in which the presence or absence of mental illness is of considerably more importance than the health or safety of the patient or protection of others in coming to decisions.

Clarity and Wide Versus Narrow Interpretations

The 1983 Act - although like its predecessor the 1959 Act emphasising a treatment model - clearly attempted to reduce the predominance of medical power in the compulsory admission and treatment of mentally disordered patients. This is most obvious in two respects: the enhanced powers and duties of social workers through the ASW role, and the use of Mental Health Review Tribunals, particularly in relation to the patient's right to legal representation and legal aid.

However, the wording of the Act in relation to health or safety of the patient or the protection of others is extremely loose, while at the same time concealing complex criteria used in practice to section people.

These loose criteria were no doubt intended to encourage judgement and flexibility in complex and sometimes crisis situations. It clearly expects the professionals to act in good faith and with reasonable care (Section 139). However, instead of encouraging flexibility and sound judgement, these criteria are frequently a charter for idiosyncratic decision-making. Thus noticeable inconsistencies exist - some people are admitted in apparently identical circumstances to others who are not - while some patients are admitted without any clear indication of the perceived possible outcome if admission does not occur (the danger). Furthermore, the looseness of the criteria allows for very different situations to lead to admission: family separation or the reputation of public figures stand alongside possible death as grounds for admission.

This width may account in part for the inconsistencies that exist. Some ASWs may adhere to a narrow interpretation of the 'health or safety of the patient' or 'protection of others' which may include injury, death or serious physical ill health - perhaps likely to be permanently disabling. Others may adhere to a wide interpretation, which will go far beyond these factors, through mental health, emotional distress, temporary damage to a child's emotional development or even inconveniencing and disturbing neighbours. Between the narrow and wide interpretations lie intermediate positions which may be adopted.

However, some inconsistencies are individual. Particular ASWs may occasionally admit patients in similar circumstances to others whom they do not admit. This again may relate to the lack of analytic clarity.

In this situation, two elements are significant:

1. *Orientation* - mental health versus social risk.

2. *Interpretation* - wide versus narrow.

If we are to take civil rights seriously (acting in good faith and with reasonable care) and balance effectively medical power, both of which are intentions of the Act, it is necessary for the ASW to take a social risk orientation; which will balance the mental health orientation more prevalent amongst doctors. In order to achieve this it is necessary to develop workable criteria to help the ASW make clearly thought-out decisions, and to contribute usefully to the training process for ASWs. In short, we need some kind of 'knowledge base' for ASW assessment of the health or safety of the patient or the protection of others.

The primary aims of increasing clarity and encouraging comprehensive exploration may have a secondary effect. Once the ASW is clearer about the precise reasons for admission it is quite possible that the *range* (narrow to wide) of interpretations will become narrower and less inconsistent. This is based on an expectation that actually identifying the danger, assessing its seriousness and the level of risk will make the precise degree of overall risk much clearer. The details of this process are outlined later. Certainly, the vagaries evident from the research contributed to a wide interpretation of risk and some degree of inconsistency. Clearer assessment may well, for example, help reduce 'admissions by default', and force the ASW to decide whether this *particular* danger in these *particular* circumstances is sufficient to justify admission. By narrowing the range of interpretations, patients may be seen to be treated with greater justice and fairness.

Providing a Social Science Knowledge Base

The approach to knowledge development adopted here falls broadly into a tradition which regards social workers as 'technicians' rather than 'helpers': where social work is seen to progress less as an art (England, 1986) than through the development of techniques based on rational analysis. This tradition has been widely espoused and is evident in much social work writing (Reid, 1978; Hoghughi, 1980a; Sheldon, 1983).

It has developed in response to two related issues: the perceived problems of social work, and the need to develop, as far as possible, a systematic knowledge base for social work. Hoghughi (1980b) suggests that many of the afflictions of social work - lack of clarity, disputed effectiveness and questionable public esteem - are self-induced:

> 'The protagonists of social work are likely to present an idealised image of it which bears little resemblance to the limitations and stresses under which social workers operate.'

Likewise, Sheldon (1983) comments that social workers, 'are rarely able to learn from mistakes as they go on'. He thinks this is partly due to the separation of two major realms of social work: an 'academic subculture', emphasising the importance of research, rational analysis and evaluation, and a 'practice subculture' suspicious of the relevance and results of research, and adhering primarily to experiential 'practice' knowledge (Sheldon, 1978).

This can lead to a state of despair about relating 'theory' to 'practice'. Davies (1985) has effectively advocated marginalising social science knowledge on the grounds that there is little evidence to suggest it has any impact on social work effectiveness, and that sociology teaching in particular may undermine and demoralise social work students. Howe

(1980) would not be surprised at this. He points to the contradictory and conflicting assumptions about humans and society which make social science knowledge ill-suited to applied work. He suggests that the continued interest in social science knowledge is a matter of homophonics - that both 'social work' and 'social science' sound as if they are related - rather than an understanding of the real properties of each. However, their positions have been hotly disputed (Hardiker, 1981; Sibeon, 1982; Sheppard, 1984); and principles have been suggested (Sheppard, 1984; Sheldon, 1978) for applying social science knowledge more systematically.

Some of the more well known technical approaches to the development of a useful social work method or knowledge base include task-centred work, the problem profile approach and the use of single case experimental designs (Reid, 1978; Hoghughi, 1980a; Sheldon, 1983). These emphasise the need for being systematic and developing coherent classifications which 'have a number of advantages over traditional forms of discussive narrative recording, in which the practitioner puts down pretty well what he chooses' (Reid, 1978).

Overall these approaches have some common tendencies:

1. They accept that there is a knowledge base, or potential knowledge base, which may be applied to practice.

2. The client is seen as the repository of a number of different qualities, which are classified.

3. There is a certain degree of detachment required - contrasting with involvement in relationships - in assessing, planning, carrying out and evaluating work.

4. It tends to be non-egalitarian: the professional 'owns' the knowledge even when it is only knowledge of method, such as task-centred work.

5. The client is perceived not so much as seeking some kind of 'spiritual rejuvenation' (Keith-Lucas, 1972) but rather as the possessor of particular problems.

6. The relationship is not perceived to be a central element of the knowledge base, although it is accepted that this can be important in engaging the client to resolve their problems.

These qualities, it should be noted, are tendencies rather than hard and fast rules. Equally, they do not preclude humanist elements such as intention, motivation and meaning (Berger and Luckman, 1966). Classifications which are developed do so within particular theoretical frameworks which do not prevent differing constructions of situations (Sheppard, 1984). Furthermore it does not preclude the use of relationships through which problems may be confronted. Indeed, it is arguable that the openness of the worker, and joint involvement with the client in tackling problems in task-centred work, would foster trust and better relationships.

Praxis in Compulsory Admission Assessment

'Praxis' refers to a situation where theory and practice are brought together. The technician approach, guided by direct research, is particularly useful in this respect. It has already been demonstrated that nebulous assessment may take place, and inconsistencies occur in practice. The law itself is vague, and encourages individualised interpretation (Hoggett, 1984). The technical approach provides the basis for a balance to the extensive knowledge available on the classification and diagnosis of mental disorder, which is likely to encourage emphasis on the mental health aspects to the detriment of the health or safety of the patient or protection of others aspects of compulsory admission assessment. Furthermore it provides a vehicle through which information gained from research about the situations ASWs confronted may be transmitted into a practice knowledge base.

This notion of praxis is something of a holy grail for social work. Its essential element is that it should be focussed on the problems confronted by social workers and their own perceived needs in terms of information to assess and resolve the problems. Thus, if we are concerned with juvenile delinquents, then useful research is that which focusses *directly on* juvenile delinquents. If there are limits to the levels at which social workers may intervene - for example, intervention at the level of social structure is beyond the bounds of legitimate practice (Howe, 1979; Galper, 1975) - then explanatory models which require amelioration of structural problems are of little use.

Thus, a necessary accompaniment to a technical approach to social work practice in this area, and for praxis to be achieved, are theoretical assumptions which are essentially oriented towards consensus. In essence, this involves general acceptance of what is or is not acceptable behaviour, and directs attention both in explanation and practice away from social structure. This fits both with law and social work practice. In fact there is an obvious link here because the social work role is, in this area, determined by the law. In adhering to a construction of problems which are defined as 'health' problems (hence the title the Mental Health Act) the law is clearly identifying its concerns as issues of deviance, with which it is appropriate that designated professionals deal. Social workers, in this area, operate very much as 'gatekeepers', defining individuals in a way that may contribute at times towards secondary deviance.

The research provides the basis for praxis because it tackles the issues in terms of the way the social workers *themselves* accounted for their actions. It draws on information, therefore, which is explicitly within a practice frame of reference. Furthermore, the legal framework requires the ASW (or nearest relative) and doctors *rather than the patient* to judge whether there are dangers to the health or safety of the patient or others need protecting. In this way the Act emphasises the importance of *attributed problems* - in this case problems attributed to the patient by the assessors - rather than *acknowledged problems* - those acknowledged by the patient themselves (Reid, 1978). Patients may deny they are mentally ill, but this will not prevent compulsory admission when considered appropriate by the doctor, ASW or nearest relative.

If 'attributed problems' are significant then it is the ASW's perception rather than the patient's which is crucial. Appropriate classification of these problems arises from within the ASW's frame of reference, but allows the ASWs at the same time to become more systematic in making their judgements.

However, this praxis does not take the form of a fully structured questionnaire. This is because the issue of assessment is not *exclusively* one of appropriate classification but also one of rational and systematic analysis. Some issues are not simply a matter of deciding what is the exact hazard or danger, but of what should be examined to establish the seriousness of danger or level of risk. This often involves questions of evidence, vulnerability, supports and so on. Hence the approach should be regarded as systematic, involving some classification, rather than exclusively classificactory.

Hazards

Dangers occur, or become more likely, in the face of particular hazards. Logically, hazards are present before or at the same time as dangers. The hazard, furthermore, will often be the most obvious factor confronting the ASW. They often need to surmise the danger from the hazard. Thus an elderly confused person wandering about during the night in winter could be a situation confronting an ASW. From this they may infer particular dangers: physical ill health, injury or possibly death.

It is appropriate, therefore, to consider hazards first. The critical area justifying admission, as we shall see, is danger. However, the hazard explains *why* the danger exists. Through the identification of hazards it is clearer why the ASW fears particular dangers, and helps to indicate in any particular case whether a danger is legitimately feared. It would, for example, take an extensive chain of reasoning, to say the least, to link the hazard of irresponsible financial management with the danger of death. By being clear about the exact nature of the hazard, therefore, the ASW begins systematically the process of considering the seriousness of the danger and level of risk.

The first classification (see Appendix to this chapter) is that of hazards. This contains the largest number of individual categories. This is perhaps because of the wide variety of circumstances which may be considered hazardous. The classification, however, emphasises the essentially *social* nature of the health or safety of the patient or protection of others. All of them involve forms of behaviour, many involve social relationships, and all relate to values.

The individual hazards are categorised within six broad domains. The first, *health,* is self-explanatory. The second, *failure to provide basic needs* , refers to those basic biological requirements to sustain an adequate life. What constitutes 'adequate', of course, is normative, and may vary between different societies and different times, but the hazards refer to areas such as lack of warmth, food, and drink. *Threatening violence* involves hazards where by action or verbal communication possible future violence is indicated. The fourth area, *actual violence* , involves violence already occurring when the ASW makes their assessment. The damage, such as personal injury, may not have occurred, but the patient's behaviour - for example having punched someone - places the person at risk of future injury. If damage had already occurred there would be a fear of further injury. The fifth area, *out of control of self and actions,* refers to a state where, without threatening or being violent, the patient is not aware of possible deleterious consequences of what they are doing, for example they have little traffic awareness, or they are confused, or have an unrealistic assessment of their own abilities. The final area refers to the *contravention of social regulations or expectations,* such as breaking the law, creating a disturbance, or inability to carry out a significant role area, such as neglect of the child caring role.

These are broad domains for guiding the ASW, and there are some overlaps. Thus, for example, it is possible for someone out of control of themselves or their actions to contravene social regulations by breaking the law (for example by wandering along the hard shoulder of a motorway). They do, however, provide a way of grouping a wide diversity of hazards. Furthermore, they are normative: what, for example, constitutes a 'social expectation' depends on the standards prevalent at the time. This is not surprising in view of the normative basis of ASW judgements.

Although hazards and dangers are - to be comprehensible - necessarily linked, a particular hazard may potentially lead to more than one danger. Thus, for example, hyperactive behaviour may make the patient more vulnerable to ill health, or become emotionally traumatic for a carer or create a relapse in mental health in a vulnerable relative (Vaughn and Leff, 1976). The outcome will depend on the circumstances in which the hazards take place.

Furthermore, there are inevitable issues of judgement. Whether or not failure to take prescribed medication constitutes a hazard relates to the imputed danger. Medication may be for relatively mild problems - cold or flu for example - or for something more serious such as pneumonia. Thus there are a number of issues to be considered after the hazard is identified before making any judgement.

Danger

Danger is best conceptualised following the work of Brown and Harris (1978) in terms of threat. This is useful in three respects. First, it is forward looking: the situation is such that there is a threat of some damage occurring in the future. Second, it is related to the hazard - it is the hazard that creates the threat of damage. Finally, it involves an element of probability: if someone is threatened with some danger it is not certain that this danger will occur - the *degree* of threat indeed is an issue related to hazard and links danger to the level of risk.

The danger is the possible feared outcome which arises in the face of the hazard. The criteria of the 'health or safety of the patient' or 'protection of others' is most comprehensible in terms of danger rather than hazard or risk, since it is the possible outcome which must be of central concern. The type of hazard or level of risk only gain significance in relation to some feared outcome. It is most useful, therefore, to consider danger in relation to the categories of the Act as follows:

1. Projected health threat - mental or physical - to the patient.

2. Projected safety threat to the patient.

3. Projected threat to others (from what should they be protected?).

Danger will be evaluated in terms of its *seriousness*. This involves:

1. Identifying the nature of the danger.

2. Identifying those vulnerabilities which may predispose the person to danger.

Mental Health Threat (Appendix 1, Classification 2). This is perhaps the most problematic area. It is included because the Mental Health Act Commission (1987) advise unequivocally that this be included as an aspect of the 'health or safety of the patient' criteria, despite being part also of the 'mental disorder' criteria. However, it raises as many questions as it answers, offering a licence to admit on mental health grounds alone, and rendering the health or safety of the patient or protection of others criteria superfluous when it is adopted. Clearly, further guidance is required: either in terms of the circumstances under which the 'mental health' criteria is appropriate, or to eliminate it completely from the health or safety of the patient or protection of others criteria. In the next chapter suggestions will be made for dealing with this issue around the concept of social functioning. However, as the Mental Health Act Commission do not specifically refer to this, it is inappropriate at this stage to incorporate it with the assessment schedule.

In view of this, it is perhaps best, first, to identify the areas broadly, according to the most recent International Classification of Diseases (World Health Organisation,1977) as follows:

                1. Neurotic
                2. Psychotic
                3. Organic Psychotic

The research indicated that, in those cases studied at least, it was psychotic conditions which exclusively fitted this criterion. If this is the intention of the Commission, then this broad division is crucial. However, further divisions may be made in terms of psychiatric diagnosis, which is the second classification identified. I assume the ASW will have some mental health knowledge, as is required, and that detailed explanation of each category is unnecessary. However, sufficient is known about the behaviour of patients when subject to these conditions to help guide the ASWs in their decision-making. The individual categories are not exhaustive, but represent those disorders most frequently seen by social workers.

Nonetheless, these divisions may be accompanied by questions which may usefully be asked by the ASW. These revolve around the central questions: is the nature of the mental illness such that compulsory admission is justified? This is quite significant. Community studies now consistently show that a high proportion of the general population suffers neurotic disorders such as anxiety or depression (Goldberg and Huxley, 1980; Henderson, Byrne and Duncan-Jones, 1981; Brown and Harris, 1978). Likewise, a considerable proportion of the elderly suffer from dementia, which may be helped, but not cured, by suitable medication (Gilleard, 1984). If, therefore, large numbers of mentally ill people (using clear medical definitions) live in the community without being even assessed for compulsory admission, then we cannot expect a person to be sectioned in all circumstances where they are mentally ill. Likewise, ASWs do not always section mentally ill patients when they - using their own definitions - do not consider them a 'danger to themselves or others'. Indeed, even some psychotic patients were not sectioned. Clearly, in some circumstances, the definition of 'health or safety' precludes some states of mental illness.

When considering admission on mental health grounds alone, certain questions may be helpful.

1. Is it a problem which is organically or psycho-socially caused? If it is the latter, then it may be possible to manipulate the environment in such a way that pressures are taken off the patient, without recourse to admission.

2. Is it a problem which may be resolved without medication? Some problems - life crises for example - may not *always* require medication ultimately to be resolved. Others, such as florid schizophrenia, require mediation (anti-psychiatric claims notwithstanding).

3. What are the likely consequences if medication is not taken? In some cases the ASW may fear a serious deterioration of the patient's condition. If this is the case the ASW may feel medical intervention is appropriate to *prevent* deterioration. This is still more emphatic if failure to treat is not only likely to lead to deterioration, but may have permanent consequences - that the condition may, for example, move from acute to chronic. Such judgements may be difficult to make, particularly so in the absence of an approved doctor (possible with Section 4), unless the ASW is very experienced in mental health.

4. Is further deterioration likely regardless of the need for medication? In some cases mental health may be likely to deteriorate in the face of existing circumstances. In these situations the environment is such that the patient would benefit from separation from overwhelming problems. A woman may, for example, be depressed following the death of a parent, live in poor housing conditions, be in financial difficulties and have difficult child care responsibilities. Such a combination may be grinding her down into deepening depression. Although environmental intervention may be the ultimate answer, admission may give this woman asylum - a respite which may prevent further deterioration by taking her out of a stressful situation.

5. Does the problem appear stable and difficult to shift? Where a patient is already suffering a mental disorder and is unlikely to change this may be indicated by a current mental health state which has been present for some time, or a chronic condition in which this episode is a relapse. Of course, the other side of this is that if the mental ill health is stable the patient may have managed perfectly well in the community for some time. Alternatively, however, the patient's social functioning may have deteriorated while the mental ill health was stable: prolonged absence from work, increasing financial hardship, social withdrawal and growing social isolation, growing indebtness, possible eviction and so on (Weissman and Paykel, 1974; Corney, 1984).

Although not strictly vulnerability factors - which may be construed as specific existing weakness in the face of which the illness danger becomes more serious - they are issues clearly associated with the mental health condition of the patient. They may, as supplementary factors, play a role in relation to mental health which is similar to that of the vulnerability factors which will be identified in relation to physical ill health. Like vulnerability factors, they provide reasons for being more concerned about the health condition of the patient.

On the basis of those factors - the nature of the mental illness, its cause, requirements for treatment and possibility of deterioration - we can rate the severity of the mental health problem which can inform the decision of whether or not to admit (see Appendix 1, Classification 2(5)).

Physical Health Threat (Appendix 1, Classification 3). This is perhaps less problematic than mental health, since it represents criteria clearly separate from mental disorder. There is, however, a wide variety of health problems - currently hundreds of diseases and syndromes exist. Furthermore, ASWs cannot pretend to medical expertise and it seems, therefore, inappropriate for the ASW to consider these in terms of detailed diagnosis.

However, it is nonetheless necessary for the ASW to obtain some idea of the severity of the ill health problem. Although, for example, a person may be ill with a common cold, this is not a condition an ASW would normally, if ever, consider sufficiently serious to justify sectioning. The ASW will obviously rely on medical advice, particularly in areas of doubt, but they will still need to consider for themselves - a *logical* necessity if they are to be agents at all independent of doctors - in the light of medical advice, the severity of the illness. A seven fold classification for physical health severity has been developed (Appendix 1, Classification 3).

Although the categories in this classification use two criteria - in some (c, d, e) they are a property of treatment, while in others they are a property of the illness - they do provide a way of considering in descending order the seriousness of the illness. However, these can only be guides. There is little question about severity in relation to categories a, b and g. However, in other areas the issue is less clear. First, it is possible that the condition which required specialist outpatient treatment may be less serious than one being treated by the GP. Indeed referral to specialists may depend upon a GP's own areas of interest or their personal attitude to referral on to others (Raynes, 1980). Second, the severity of an illness treated by a particular group can vary: an opthalmologist may see someone for a relatively minor eye irritation or for a disease which threatens his sight. Third, even when an illness is transient - possibly influenza - it legally justifies admission, and the ASW must consider whether admitting on this basis constitutes an acceptable interpretation. Overall, there is a *tendency* to increased seriousness as the patient first requires the GP, then outpatient, then in-patient specialist treatment, and it provides a framework through which the ASW can make more considered judgements. This is consistent with Section 13(2) where the ASW is expected to 'consider all the circumstances of the case', which in the memorandum specifically includes medical opinion (DHSS, 1983).

The term 'consider' is important here, because this clearly indicates that the ASW is not expected slavishly to follow medical judgement but to subject that judgement to examination before reaching a decision.

A further issue is that of vulnerabilities. Do any exist which are likely to exacerbate the physical ill health (Classification 3:2)? The first two categories here involve the issue of frailty. Frailty refers to general weakness or low resistance in a person which may affect their ability to combat an ill health problem. This is particularly obvious in some elderly people who simply because of age may find it difficult to resist ill health. Thus a chest infection which might be a minor irritant to an able bodied young adult may be potentially life threatening to a frail elderly person.

A specific physical illness which the patient already has may be a further complicating factor. A person with multiple sclerosis (MS) may be at a relatively mild or early stage, or be going through a period of remission. An attack of influenza, which for most people might only lead to a few days in bed, may well be considerably more serious for the MS sufferer. They may develop, for example, respiratory complications, or have a relapse in their MS symptoms.

Others may be weakened or 'run down' through specific causes, for example they may be going through a manic phase, becoming increasingly active and having little sleep, which may leave them more and more exhausted. In that stage of exhaustion they may be far more vulnerable in the face of any particular illness. The same, finally, might be said in relation to environmental vulnerabilities. Someone living, for instance, in a damp or inadequately heated house may be considerably more at risk as a result of a viral or other infection. A patient may have one or more of these vulnerabilities. Certainly where more than one exists the ASW may feel they have an 'additive' effect - that is they increase the patient's vulnerability to the particular illness which is of concern.

The extent of vulnerability is assessed in terms of its *significance.* This is a function of two elements: relevance and degree of vulnerability. Vulnerability itself gains its importance in terms of its *interaction* with the health threat - that is, the health threat becomes more severe in the face of the existing vulnerability. If a vulnerability is to have an effect on the health threat it must first of all be relevant. The MS identified as a vulnerability in one of the previous examples was significant in part because it was likely to work with the influenza to have a greater impact on the patient's health than if the MS were not present. Other factors - a sprained ankle for example - would not be expected to interact with the influenza and hence would not be relevant. This leads to the second element - the degree of vulnerability. The relevant vulnerability may have a greater or lesser impact on the health threat. In the case of the MS there would be a possibility that it would have a considerable impact, although, of course, the ASW would assess this in terms of the particular circumstance he confronts and in the light of medical advice.

Hence, when the ASW rates the significance of a vulnerability, they must first be clear that it is relevant and then estimate its likely impact on the health threat. This relationship between threat and vulnerability factors is applicable to other areas of the patient's safety and protection of others, which will be discussed later.

Safety Threat (Appendix 1, Classification 4). As with health dangers, the interpretation of what constitutes a threat to the patient's safety is not clear, and depends on whether a wide or narrow interpretation is followed. Few would disagree with the inclusion of possible death or injury as safety threats, although even with the latter the injury may be mild (some bruising) or severe (broken bones) and these may be judged differently in relation to admission. Other circumstances relating to the physical integrity of the patient, such as rape or sexual assault, would also be relatively uncontroversial. However, these alone would constitute a narrow interpretation of safety. If further circumstances were to be included a wider interpretation is necessary. While Hoggett (1984) accepts this wider interpretation to be within the meaning of the Act, Anderson-Ford and Halsey (1984) do not.

The issue of safety can be considered in terms of the threat of loss. This can be divided broadly into three domains: physical (for example injury, i.e. loss of physical integrity), loss of social relationships, which may have emotional implications, and material loss, such as financial or employment. These are shown in Classification 4. Although the categories are fairly wide, their relevance will depend upon a wide or narrow interpretation of the law. Certainly, the research indicated some ASWs were interpreting the Act quite widely: hence the admission of the manic man open to financial exploitation because of his 'immense generosity', while in other cases possible separation from the family was suggested which may be classified either as safety of the patient or the protection of others, since both are centrally involved.

These dangers are sufficiently wide that *vulnerabilities* are best considered not as a separate classification, but as related to specific areas. Each category may carry a number of possible vulnerabilities which are extremely variable. Thus, for example, loss of children may be a greater threat where the patient is a single parent with no one else to provide necessary support for the child. Likewise, loss of employment may be more likely where the patient has a poor relationship with the employer, or where the firm is looking to make redundancies.

Protection of Other Persons (Appendix 1, Classification 5). The protection of other persons is the last of the danger issues identified in the Act. The issue here is: from what are the other persons being protected? In some respects this might at first be seen as a mirror image of the 'safety of the patient' - for we are here concerned about the threat to the safety of other people. However, the categories which may be identified yield factors which go beyond this mirror image (Classification 5).

It is clear that issues of health (mental or physical) may be included. However, a very wide interpretation allows the ASW to go beyond these factors included in health or safety of the patient, involving, for example, emotional trauma, or even intrusive behaviour. Hoggett (1984) comments, in relation to protection of others, that:

> 'The only confident statement is that the protection of property alone is not enough'.

Jones (1988) considers the interpretation of 'protection of others' should be limited to emotional trauma, not extending in our terminology to intrusive behaviour or offending public taste.

Even when a wide interpretation is taken, it is incumbent on the ASW, as with other areas, to consider whether the problem in any individual category is sufficiently serious to merit compulsory admission. Death is self evidently serious. However, in all other areas an assessment of severity is necessary. This is even the case in an area which would be considered within a narrow interpretation of the Act, physical injury. Thus, some injuries - broken bones for example - would be considered severe enough, while others - mild bruising for example - would probably not. Thus we do not simply have a variation in categories based on *wide versus narrow* interpretation, we also have an assessment of individual categories based on severity. Furthermore, of course, more than one category may be involved. Thus both emotional trauma and offending public taste may be present. An initial assessment of severity involves examining the combination of areas, and the severity of each.

The rating of severity has a further element which involves identifying who it is that requires protection, that is the *focus*. The danger to some people may be greater than to other people. A woman, elderly person or child may be more vulnerable to physical injury by a man than another man, simply because of size or strength. Likewise, a woman may present less of an injury threat to an able bodied man (unless a weapon such as a knife is used). Furthermore, there may be less patient contact with some people than others: a spouse would generally have more contact than a distant acquaintance. There would, therefore, be a variation in the *opportunity* for the danger to occur.

The final element - *vulnerability* - when assessing protection of others involves relating the particular hazard and danger to its focus - the particular person/s concerned. If for example the danger is emotional trauma to the wife, and the hazard is verbal abuse, a recent bereavement which she has suffered may make her more vulnerable to the patient's behaviour. Thus the assessment of severity of the danger depends on the nature of the danger, the type of hazard, to whom it is directed and the nature of the vulnerability. Again, therefore, rather than categorise vulnerabilities separately, it is best to consider them in terms of already identified specific dangers, asking the question whether any vulnerabilities exist in relation to those dangers and how severe they are.

Evaluating Danger: Seriousness

The central question confronting the ASW is: what are the likely consequences of failing to admit the patient? The consequences have been ordered around the classification of areas of patient's health, patient's safety and the protection of other persons, as in the Act. It is important to recognise that these areas are not mutually exclusive: it is possible both in principle and in practice for dangers to exist in all three areas at once.

From the information gained, the ASW is able to judge the *seriousness* of the danger. However, it is a mistake to make a simple correlation between the number of categories involving danger and the overall seriousness of the danger. Seriousness may be seen to be a function of a number of factors.

1. Whether a wide or narrow interpretation is taken. The latter would effectively exclude some areas from consideration.

2. The concern arising from individual categories. Some, such as possible death, will cause - one hopes - the ASW considerably more concern than offending public taste (although they may be placed under more pressure to admit by neighbours in the latter case).

3. The severity attached to the *individual* categories (as already assessed) as well as to the whole area of health *or* safety *or*

protection of others. There may, of course, be a threat in more than one area: for example a patient with an infectious disease who is not seeking medical help will not only be presenting a threat to their own health or safety, but others may well need protecting from the health risks he presents.

Further considerations involve:

4. The patient's vulnerability and supplementary mental health factors.

5. Who requires protection (protection of others) which relates to vulnerability and opportunity for threat.

In each of the three main areas - health or safety of the patient and protection of others - a simple rating system is used to indicate the severity of threat and significance of vulnerability, or in the case of mental health, the supplementary factors. These range, as shown in the Appendix, from 5 (very severe and very significant) to 1 (mild) in each of the areas of health, safety and protection of others. Although we cannot use these numbers as hard and fast indicators of when a patient should or should not be admitted - they are after all attached to *judgements* by the ASW - they have the advantage of providing a simple additive dimension whereby severity of threat and significance of vulnerability may be related.

Where these are related the ASW is trying to assess the effect of the interaction of the two factors. An elderly person living in a house slightly cold and damp may contract influenza. Both the health threat (influenza) and the vulnerability (cold and damp house) may be rated mild to moderate (in severity and significance) giving a total score of 4 - two for each category. This would give an indicator of the overall severity of the ill health threat, which when both elements are rated together would be greater than the severity of ill health when assessed alone. Although it would be wrong to provide a particular - and arbitrary - cut-off point, it is suggested here that where a total score of 4 or more is reached the ASW may need to consider carefully the need for compulsory admission (if the patient is mentally disordered and refusing admission).

However, three additional points should be made. First, as with all areas of the assessment, the rating of severity of threat and significance of vulnerability is a matter for the ASW. It is based on their judgement of the situation. However, the addition of scores will help to underline for ASWs themselves the implications of their judgements about the threat and vulnerability. Second, the system of rating the severity of threat numerically is only significant where both threat *and* vulnerability are involved. There is little need for the ASW to give the rating of 'quite severe' ill health threat a numerical value of 4 where no vulnerability is involved, because this adds nothing to their initial linguistic assessment. Third, it is not appropriate to add scores together from different areas. Thus, where a health threat, safety threat and protection of others threat each have a severity rating of mild, thus scoring 1 each, it is wrong to add them together to achieve a total rating of 3. This is because there is no interactive effect as there is between the particular danger and the vulnerability the patient has to this danger. It may well be, therefore, that where the ASW has rated the threat as mild in two or more areas they nonetheless regard the overall seriousness of the danger to be mild.

An overall rating of the danger from 'very serious' through to 'no threat' can now be made, taking into account the severity of threat and significance of vulnerability in all the main areas concerned in any particular case. This, then, provides us with one of the two main elements in compulsory assessment. For the other we must turn to the assessment of the level of risk.

Level of Risk

Risk is the concept which links hazard to danger. As in Brearley's (1982) terms, referring to the 'relative variation in possible outcomes' it is, the reader will recall, closely related to probability (that particular outcomes will occur). It is this which links particular hazards to particular dangers. The hazard is the factor which creates or increases the possibility of a particular danger occurring: if a hazard is not present, then the likelihood of the danger occurring is correspondingly reduced. To use our earlier example, it is reasonable to project that the presence of a banana peel on the pavement makes it more likely that the subject will fall and hurt themselves; without it this outcome is less likely.

The assessment of risk, therefore, should be a rational analysis based on the properties of the interacting elements. Thus the assessment of risk relating to a manic male who is verbally threatening physical violence to his wife depends on his physical capacity to inflict this violence, her relative weakness (if this is the case), his mental state - whether he is aggressive or not - his opportunity for being violent, and whether his verbal threats are just that or likely to turn into physical violence. (For example, is genuine affection likely to overcome aggression? Are these statements devoid of any real intent? Is he capable of concentrating for sufficient time on one thing to be likely to carry out these threats?)

These principles are equally applicable to compulsory admissions. Insufficient awareness of specific environmental hazards such as road traffic may lead to serious danger of injury on the part of the patient, or alternatively that in taking avoidance action other road users may be injured. Failure to take necessary medication, however, may only threaten the health of the patient rather than other people, or if the condition is infectious, will threaten other's health rather than injury.

When assessing risk rigorously, and as a consequence of the concepts and arguments so far developed, the ASW will be carrying out the following steps:

1. The identification of a hazard.

2. The identification of a particular danger.

3. Assessing the likelihood of the particular danger occurring in the face of the particular hazard.

4. Assessing the likelihood of alternative outcomes occurring in the face of the hazard.

5. Comparing this with the probability of the danger occurring had that hazard not been present.

Risk, therefore, refers to the variation in possible outcomes because, in the face of particular hazards, a projected outcome is only one of a number of possible alternatives. This is quite clear from the earlier research analysing 'level of risk' where the ASW accounts, even with their strongest evidence pointing in one particular direction (Demonstrated Danger), did not preclude *all* possibility of alternative outcomes. Different situations, for example, 'Uncertain but Dangerous' specifically included possible alternative outcomes. Hence, risk relates to the relative likelihood of alternative possible outcomes.

However, this relates also to the presence or absence of particular hazards, or the presence of alternative hazards. In each of these situations the relative likelihood of particular projected dangers occurring will vary. With a banana skin you may be more likely to slip and hurt yourself than without a banana skin. Alternatively, a cracked pavement may also present a risk of hurting yourself, but instead of slipping and pulling a muscle you might be more likely to sprain an ankle.

In doing this the ASW is:

a) Assessing the probability of a particular danger occurring in the face of a particular hazard, compared with alternative possible outcomes.

b) Assessing risk against some implicit notion of normal, acceptable risk-taking in everyday life.

This process was, in fact, carried out in the research on some of the previous examples examining ASW accounts and their assessments. It is best illustrated where some uncertainty existed about the nature of the danger. Thus, the reader will recall a schizophrenic man who had left home during the night, and was considered at risk, although he had some money and was not aggressive. The ASW was worried that:

> 'He had been wandering the street at night and the early hours of the morning and he was quite dishevelled. He was not really rational'.

The hazards are here - wandering about at night in a non-rational state - but the danger is not. We speculated that it could be a number of things - that he may be attacked or robbed, or suffer exposure, or the traffic might hit or injure him. Without some indication of what danger exists, we cannot begin to assess the increased probability of the danger occurring in the face of the hazard concerned.

Let us assume that the danger is a fear that the traffic may hit or injure him - a 'safety of the patient' danger (although it might be any one or more of these dangers, or other unstated dangers). We need first to assess the probability of this happening. This necessarily involves a number of steps.

First: Does his mental state prevent him from manifesting any 'traffic awareness'? He might not be quite rational, but he may be aware enough to negotiate the traffic.

Second: If his traffic awareness is impaired, to what extent is this the case? It might be only slightly impaired, and no worse than that of many other people - for example, an elderly person who we would not dream of sectioning. If so, does this provide us with the justification for compulsory admission? Of course his traffic awareness may be greatly impaired so that he might easily walk out straight in front of a car without looking where he was going.

Third: Is he placing himself in situations which increase the likelihood of a confrontation with traffic? If he is staying well clear of roads, especially busy ones, he is staying away from the hazard. From the account this does not seem to be the case - he is wandering about, and the ASW cannot be sure where he will go. However, he is out at night, and there is less traffic about then. Will he return home if asked, and will he stay clear of traffic during the day?

These are all questions which help the ASW judge the probability of a particular danger occurring in the face of a particular hazard - non-rational wandering. However, we have a further stage of assessment comparing the hazard with a non-hazard situation.

Fourth: What risk is there of this danger occurring if the hazard were not present? We can look at this in two ways. First, the risk may be assessed in relation to the patient's likely functioning when the hazard does not exist. This is available to the ASW, in particular, when they have previous knowledge of the patient. Second, it may be compared with the risk to the public as a whole of injury from traffic accidents. We know already that large numbers of people are injured or killed on the roads each year, yet this is perceived as a part of 'normal' risk taking.

On the basis of these questions it is possible to make some judgement of normal acceptable risk. In so doing, we are taken back to Brearley's notion of risk as the relative variations in possible outcome: a variation in the face of the hazard from the probability of the danger occurring where the patient is functioning normally, and the variation when compared with the probability of the danger occurring to others in the course of normal everyday life.

The process, which reflects the stages of analysis (1) to (5) above represents a clarification of the exact nature of the problem, and the risks attached. The ASW is thereby removed from making judgements based purely on hunch, and states more precisely the nature of the situation. This allows them to make judgements, whatever they may be, in a clearer, more cognitive and rational way.

The questions addressed in the case were particular to this example. When going through this process, however, a number of questions may be addressed which may be phrased in a way more generally applicable. These may be divided into two:

a)   Those relating to the behaviour of the person and the danger itself.

b) Those relating to social supports whose use may reduce or eliminate the danger.

Behaviour of Person and Danger

1. Is the behaviour of the person contributing to the increased probability of danger? For example, they may not be eating, or be in a confused state, and hence possibly at risk of a health or injury danger.

2. How likely are they to change their behaviour, if this is the case, as the danger becomes more manifest? For example, they may not be eating or drinking - perhaps because they are depressed, or so hyperactive they do not stop to take time to eat. If this is the case, they may, once they are hungry, take sufficient time to eat, and avert any danger of physical ill health. Alternatively, they may be sufficiently aware of their behaviour to alter it: the man in the previous example may have had sufficient insight to avoid busy roads.

3. Is the danger itself transitory or self-limiting? A person rushing about may be in danger of exhaustion. However, this may lead inevitably to rest and recovery as the person becomes too tired to continue.

4. Is the patient sufficiently in control of themselves to prevent the danger occurring? For example, someone may have limited insight into their paranoid state (voices telling them their wife is unfaithful), sufficient to prevent any harm or injury coming to her.

Social Supports

Social support assessment is critical to the analysis of risk, since the presence of social support - which, as we shall see, may potentially involve a variety of people, whether professional, familial or other informal social contacts - can reduce the level of risk in particular situations. Hence it is appropriately included in the schedule as part of the section on Level of Risk.

The central issue here is: do social supports exist which reduce the likelihood of the danger occurring? The issue is approached by drawing upon, in particular, the work of Hans Veiel (1985) who developed a conceptual framework for the examination of the components of social support. He divides the framework into a number of areas over two dimensions. The first dimension relates to *type* of support. This may be either *psychological* or *instrumental*. Psychological support comprises transactions 'aimed at changing intra-psychic parameters' such as mood, attitudes or cognitive processing: within this the emotional support may be distinguished from the more cognitive aspect of psychological support. Thus coping with stress may be undertaken by some form of cognitive work to change perceptions, or through emotional support which helps to lift mood, or cope better with that mood.

Instrumental support is support designed to help the individual's overt performance directly. This may be further divided into practical support and informational support. Informational support is provision of information which will help in relation to particular tasks, for example providing information on DSS benefits enabling the person to obtain extra financial support. Practical support is the provision of direct practical help, provided by the supporter themselves. This might, for example, involve helping a disabled person with shopping or obtaining their DSS benefits.

Veiel further distinguishes between everyday and crisis support: this refers to the nature of the problem focus. Is the support to get someone over a crisis or is it more broadly, socially integrative transactions? This has a temporal aspect: 'socially integrative transactions' basically refer to social relationships which have an everyday and permanent quality about them; for example, friendship. These may be expected to be relatively stable over time. Attitudes such as felt security and self-esteem may consequently be expected: thus continued social support may lead to personality characteristics which may have more immediate beneficial effects than the social transactions themselves. Alternatively there may be a long-term need for instrumental support, such as practical support required by a physically handicapped person. Social integration may be regarded as promoting mental health by making individuals more robust and better able to bear stressful experiences in general. Crisis support, on the other hand, is aimed at coping with - by directly reducing the impact of - specific crises and stressors. These may, for example, be bereavement, in which emotional support is offered, or financial in the case of a financial crisis. Again, these may be instrumental or psychological, but relate to the particular crisis rather than the long-term need for social interaction.

The second dimension is the *relational context*. This refers to the general role relationship between the support provider and recipient within which supportive transactions take place. This source of support may, first, be 'natural support providers' (informal supports) - people whose function is not *primarily* to give support to other people with their problems. These may, for example, be relatives, friends or workmates.

The second source of support is that of institutional, professional or voluntary providers (formal supports) whose purpose is the provision of support. Obvious examples of this support group include social workers, doctors, nurses or voluntary befrienders. The *type* of support provided is not dependent on which group provides it. Thus it is possible in principle for natural support providers to supply psychological or instrumental support as it is for formal supports.

Two further issues arise which cut across the two main dimensions. The first relates to the what is needed/who should provide it distinction. It may, for example, be as important to identify who can best provide the support as the type of support required. For example, the *quality* of the relationship may be critical in determining its utility in alleviating the problem. A well known example is that of 'intimacy' - a close supportive relationship with spouse or partner - which Brown and Harris (1978) found protected against the onset of depression. Other kinds of support, from friends or relatives, were not found to have the same protective quality in relation to the psychological support needs of women. Clearly, the different support providers are not always interchangeable in relation to the specific type of support needs of an individual.

The second issue relates to the difference between the amount of support received and the adequacy of this support. An individual may be receiving support from a number of people, but may not find this adequate to their needs: as with women who in the face of factors provoking depression do not have a close intimate relationship, even if they have affective support from other people. In other cases, the amount of support, such as practical support required by a handicapped person, may be more closely related to its adequacy. These various dimensions, and social support in general, are of some significance in the assessment. A person who is failing to eat on their own - for example an elderly demented person - may nevertheless be prepared to eat when supervised by a relative, friend, voluntary or professional helper. The risk of self harm by a person who has suffered recent and serious loss will be reduced if someone is on hand to 'keep an eye on them' and give them practical and emotional support.

Three initial questions arise: What type of support is required? What type of support is available? Who can provide this support? These supports can usefully be shown diagramatically in terms of types and providers.

	Types	Providers	
		Formal	Informal
Psychological	Cognitive Affective	A	B
Instrumental	Information Practical	C	D

This division can be illustrated fairly simply. Thus, for example, social services may provide meals on wheels or occupational therapy aids (Formal-Instrumental) or counselling and emotional support (Formal-Psychological/Affective). Likewise, a neighbour may provide help with cleaning the house to ensure standards of hygiene (Informal-Instrumental) or a relative may offer emotional comfort following the death of a spouse (Informal/Psychological/Affective).

The important point here is the matching of the *support need* with the *support provision.* There is little point giving emotional support to someone who is in danger because of standards of hygiene! It is, therefore, necessary to identify what support is required and who it is who can provide it. This may relate, first, to the quality of the relationship previously identified. Thus on some occasions an intimate relationship may be most significant. In the absence of such an intimate relationship it may not matter greatly whether the support is provided informally through friends, or formally, through counsellors, social workers or befrienders (except perhaps where particular psychological skills are required).

Clearly, overall the ASW may look to formal or informal supports. A critical factor is availability, and as Bowl, Barnes and Fisher (1987) point out, there is a distinct lack of formal community supports as alternatives to hospital admission. However, this should not prevent the ASW examining the availability of informal supports, where appropriate, which may even be brought together in the form of a 'care plan' combining formal and informal supports enabling the person to remain in the community. Thus an elderly demented person, risking their health or life through failure to eat and inadequate hygiene, may be helped perhaps by home help and meals on wheels (formal supports), plus more frequent visits by neighbours and relatives who will check on the safety of the person, provide other meals as required (for example at weekends) and respond flexibly to needs as they arise. This may be achieved through a clearly timetabled care plan, outlining the participants' responsibilities. Additionally a social worker may make periodic assessment visits to monitor the situation, and keep in touch with support providers. In this way a possible crisis may be turned into a form of preventive action.

The dimensions of social support can be examined through Classification 6 (Appendix 1). If providers of the requisite support needs exist, then two further questions arise:

1. What capacity do they have to provide sufficient support to reduce the risk to an acceptable level?

2. Will they be able to sustain the support for a sufficiently long time?

This depends on the temporal aspect of the support required: is the need primarily for crisis support or for longer-term integrative transactions? Although the situation may be quite serious it may possibly be transient as a result of a crisis. A patient may feel depressed and suicidal if they have lost their spouse and child in a car accident. In another case longer-term support may be in the form of the supervision of medication required by a patient. The length of time required for support can have an impact on the adequacy of the support, as can the *intensity* of support required over the relevant period of time.

A home help may, for example, be able to provide home management support, but this may not be sufficient to provide for all the patient's requirements. If their perceived need is for personal supervision, they may simply not be able to devote enough time to the tasks required to support the patient adequately. Likewise, a relative volunteering to monitor the patient's behaviour may live too far away to do so effectively; it may not be easy to get to the patient's house, and responding flexibly to his needs may be very difficult. Furthermore, the capacity to *sustain* that support is important. A physically frail person may be able to help with personal and home hygiene for a while, but this may be beyond them in the longer term. Likewise, a nurse's ability to provide the required nursing care will depend on other demands being placed on them if the needs last over some time, and on the extent of the patient's needs. Hence, in addition to the issues of the support required, support available and who can provide this support, there is also the question of whether the support is adequate.

The Evaluation of Evidence

The final area of relevance is the evaluation of evidence. In certain respects this has been considered already. Much of the work involved in assessing the level of risk requires examining closely evidence brought forward to establish the severity of danger or level of risk: thus it is not sufficient simply to state that a person is wandering and irrational and therefore at risk in traffic but it is necessary to examine this statement with considerably greater precision. However, further criteria can be identified:

1. How comprehensive is the information being collected?

2. How reliable is the information provided?

These criteria - comprehensiveness and reliability - are widely applicable to social work assessments. This is the case with, however, provisos in relation to section assessments.

Given the civil rights implications of these assessments, the need for comprehensiveness is obvious. This is recognised in the DHSS (1983) *Memorandum* in relation to the duty to 'interview in a suitable manner'. Furthermore, the more comprehensive (relevant) information obtained, the better the foundation for good judgement. Although some situations will be sufficiently clearcut to make decisions based only on an interview with the patient, ideally this would involve, where possible, interviews with other relevant individuals - relatives, friends, involved professionals and so on. This would enhance the ASW's ability to place the patient's behaviour in its social context, allowing better understanding of the influence of their behaviour on others, of others' behaviour on them (Is the patient, for example, the one with the problems, or is he the weak link in a family with problems?), the extent to which mitigating supports exist and the extent to which the behaviour differs from their normal behaviour. This may not be possible, at least with such thoroughness, when interviewing the patient alone. These are all areas which - as has been discussed - help assess the level of risk. The assessment schedule deals with this by requiring the ASW to indicate those who can provide useful information, and those whom they *actually* interview. This will indicate the extent to which they have contacted relevant individuals. It may not always be possible to identify clearly those whom it is most important to interview. However, in some cases it may be obvious - where, for example, the police have picked the patient up in a public place, or a relative or friend lives with them.

The other main issue is that of reliability. Always important, the specific circumstances of compulsory admissions make this particularly difficult. Two important elements are here. First, the truthfulness of accounts may be problematic. Most patients, as shown by figures on the distribution of compulsory and informal admissions, are not delighted by the prospect of hospital admission - hence those which are compulsory. Thus there may be attempts to deny or cover up hazardous behaviour or to avoid discussing aspects of their mental illness which may present a potential threat (e.g. suicidal feelings). Likewise relatives, who are very often under the most pressure from the patients, very often have a stake in getting the patient admitted, which may well affect their description of the hazards presented by the patient.

Accuracy is the other problematic area. Like the lawyer, the ASW may usefully distinguish between behaviour *seen* by the person interviewed, and that which is hearsay. Although stated in good faith, hearsay, because of the 'chain' of reporting, gives greater scope for inaccuracy and distortion. The same may apply to the GP reporting the view of others who have seen the patient's behaviour.

Another aspect of accuracy is that of professional - particularly medical - advice. This is the case, for example, where claims are being made about likely hazards related to particular mental or physical ill health. This is not a matter of disputing medical judgement, which the ASW is not competent to do (except perhaps, for example in GPs' assessments of mental health) (Bean, 1980). They are, however, through judicious questioning, able to help the doctor consider clearly whether the hazards giving rise to concern actually apply in a particular case.

Overall, then, two elements are necessary when analysing evidence:

1. The critical analysis of evidence presented to assess whether the claims presented are justified.

2. The collection of sufficient information to be as confident as practicable that the information gleaned is clear and accurate.

Although section assessments are sometimes crisis situations, this is not always the case, so the ASW should not unnecessarily experience them this way. Section 4, which is the 'crisis section', is only relevant where admission is of 'urgent necessity' and obtaining a second doctor would involve 'undesirable delay'. With Sections 2, 3 and 7, five clear days can elapse *between* the days of the separate medical assessments (Section 12(1)). If the ASW does not see the section assessment as a discrete single interview situation - which he does not need to do - this gives the opportunity to conduct a piece of short-term work, monitoring the patients and collecting further information, contributing to a more informed decision.

The ASW's behaviour may reflect their orientation rather than the patient's circumstances or the requirements of law. Huntington (1981) contrasts the 'action' orientation of medicine - a belief embedded in medical culture that it is important to act quickly to avert possible serious consequences - and the 'holding' orientation of social work - a belief that it is important to consider situations carefully before taking hasty actions which may be ill judged or harmful. In the case of compulsory admissions, the very proximity of social work to the medical domain may lead to the unnecessary acquisition of an 'action' orientation, particularly if pressed by relatives, neighbours and doctors. This does not mean that speedy action is not at times required, rather it emphasises further the need for the ASW's behaviour to fit in with the broader attitudes, values and knowledge base of social work as a whole.

The Assessment of Overall Risk

The ASW is now in a position to provide the complementary dimension to the seriousness of danger: the level of risk. Such an assessment can be based broadly around two areas.

1. Factors creating the danger: here we are concerned with the nature of the hazard and its seriousness, whether or not vulnerabilities exist which would exacerbate the projected danger, who is placed at risk of the danger, whether alternative outcomes are possible and so on.

2. Factors mitigating against the danger: this involves issues such as whether the patient is capable of altering hazard inducing behaviour, the likelihood of them placing themselves in hazardous situations, and whether supports are available which render the situation less hazardous.

On the basis of this the ASW may make an assessment of overall risk ranging from high risk to low risk. It should be emphasised that this is a separate judgement to that of seriousness of danger. We may, for example, regard physical harm as a greater (more serious) danger than intrusive behaviour. Yet in one particular situation there may be a *low risk* of physical harm, while in another there is a *high risk* of intrusive behaviour. Risk and danger are conceptually separate. It would be wrong, therefore, despite the seriousness of physical harm, to regard *any* situation involving physical harm as high risk, and any situation involving intrusive behaviour as low risk. In these examples we have:

a) serious danger - low risk (physical harm)

b) mild danger - high risk (intrusive behaviour)

Decision-making in relation to particular patients can, then, be made on the basis of the *combined* assessment of seriousness of danger and level of risk. If the principles of justice are to be followed - that people should be treated equally, except in the face of relevant differences (like should be treated as like) - we should aim for a fairly narrow threshold of risk.

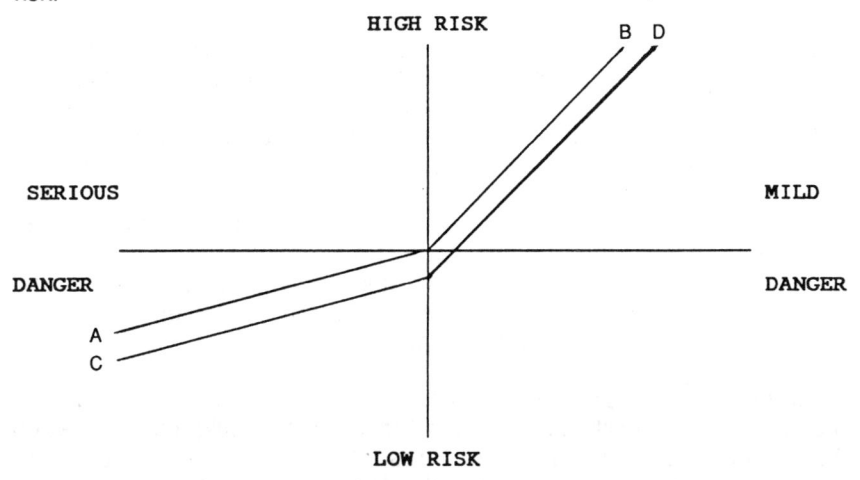

```
                    HIGH RISK       B  D
                        |          //
                        |         //
                        |        //
                        |       //
                        |      //
                        |     //
 SERIOUS                |    //                      MILD
                        |   //
                        |  //
 ─────────────────_____|_//_____
                      __/ /
 DANGER         _____/   /                          DANGER
             __/        /
        A __/          /
          _____/
        C
                        |
                        |
                    LOW RISK
```

This might be represented diagrammatically, for example, as between lines A-B and C-D. This would indicate fairly narrow boundaries, where uncertainty existed, and the patient might or might not be compulsorily admitted. The narrowness of this 'grey' area of the threshold of risk would prevent the patient's civil rights being quite so subject to the whim of the involved professionals. Certainly, the greater sensitisation of ASWs to the complexity of analysis, together with appropriate categories through which stricter definition of the situation may be made, would both aid this process, and sensitise the ASWs still further to the civil rights implications of their assessments. On its own this represents a great stride forward.

Concluding Comments

The assessment schedule is, of course, intended for use when assessing the risk to, or presented by, the mentally disordered patient. Although it may appear painstaking when first encountered by the ASW it is, as with all such schedules, one whose use will benefit from familiarity. To the extent that it is complex, furthermore, it reflects the complexity of the situation which often confronts the ASW. Certainly it provides the ASW with the opportunity to take a step-by-step approach to the assessment of possible compulsory admissions. Second, it should be remembered that although all aspects should be examined only some will be relevant in any particular situation. Hence the ASW may in some cases only be concerned about the threat to others, since no threat to the health or safety of the patient will be apparent.

The schedule may also be used as a focus for training. The extensive period now required for ASW training provides the opportunity for acquainting 'trainees' with the schedule. However, it may also be used to help develop their abilities in relation to compulsory admission assessments. This may be achieved, first, through the examination of detailed case studies which would allow them to assess all the relevant aspects of those cases. When undertaken by groups of trainees, this would contribute to a more closely shared perspective of the circumstances where admissions should or should not take place. Second, it may be used when ASW 'trainees' accompany ASWs on compulsory admission assessments. This would help both trainees and ASWs examine the situation closely, and help the trainee develop an understanding of existing practice standards.

It will be evident from this that increasing use of the schedule would provide the possibility of a means for increasing alignment between ASWs on what constitutes the threshold of risk. This is because individual assessments would draw the ASW's attention to a similar range of factors to be assessed, and because it provides a systematic means for joint and group discussions between different ASWs and trainees which may enhance the consistency of assessments.

APPENDIX 1

COMPULSORY ADMISSION ASSESSMENT SCHEDULE

CLASSIFICATION 1: HAZARDS

Please indicate which of the following hazards are present.

HEALTH:
1. Failure to take prescribed medication ☐
2. Failure to seek necessary medical help ☐
3. Hyperactive behaviour (sleeplessness/ restless etc.) ☐
4. Unhygienic living conditions/personal neglect of hygiene ☐

FAILURE TO PROVIDE BASIC NEEDS:
5. Failure to eat and drink sufficiently ☐
6. Lack of gas/electricity for warmth/light ☐
7. Lack of accommodation/eviction ☐
8. Going out naked or insufficiently dressed to prevent serious personal heat loss ☐
9. Lack of money/failure to obtain money (e.g. DSS benefits) necessary to buy basic provisions ☐

THREATENING VIOLENCE:
10. Verbal abuse/angry outbursts at others short of direct threats of physical violence ☐
11. Verbally threatening others with physical violence ☐
12. Verbally threatening aggression towards property ☐
13. Actual aggression towards property ☐
14. Physical behavioural threats (e.g. waving knife at someone/ gesticulating with fist threateningly) ☐

ACTUAL VIOLENCE:
15. Actual violence (e.g. punching others which may lead to injury) ☐

OUT OF CONTROL OF SELF AND ACTIONS:	16.	Insufficient awareness of specific environmental hazards (e.g. road traffic) ☐
	17.	Patient in a generally confused state (where they are, what they are intending to do, recognition of places and people) ☐
	18.	Sexually promiscuous/irresponsible, hence open to exploitation by others* ☐
	19.	Financially unaware/irresponsible, hence open to exploitation by others ☐
	20.	Irresponsible financial management/ spending money indiscriminately ☐
	21.	Unrealistic assessment of own abilities (e.g. beliefs of physical prowess which may place them in physical danger) ☐
	22.	Persistent derogatory accusations against others which are untrue (e.g. that spouse is having an affair or is alcoholic) ☐
CONTRAVENING SOCIAL REGULATIONS OR EXPECTATIONS:	23.	Non-violent illegal behaviour/lack of awareness of legal rules (e.g. no concept of property ownership, taking objects indiscriminately, libellous statements about others) ☐
	24.	Social withdrawal/loss of contact or communication with others
	25.	Creating a disturbance or nuisance (publicly noisy, swearing etc.) ☐
	26.	Neglect of necessary sustaining/ nurturing role for dependent children ☐
OTHER:	27.	Other (specify) ☐

---

* Note that sexual deviancy or immoral conduct are excluded under Section 1 as grounds upon which a *mental disorder* may be identified in the patient. It may represent a hazard, however, which may threaten the patient's health or safety, as outlined in the research.

DANGERS

CLASSIFICATION 2: MENTAL HEALTH THREAT

Please indicate which of the following mental health dangers are present or feared.

1. BROAD CLASSIFICATION: Organic Psychotic ☐
   Psychotic ☐
   Neurotic ☐
   None ☐

2. DETAILED DIAGNOSIS:

Organic Psychotic

Senile dementia ☐
Pre senile dementia ☐
Alcoholic psychosis* ☐
Drug psychosis* ☐

Psychotic

Schizophrenia ☐
Mania/manic depressive psychosis ☐
Unipolar depressive psychosis ☐

Neurotic

Neurotic depression ☐
Alcohol dependence syndrome* ☐

Anorexia nervosa ☐
Acute stress reaction ☐
Anxiety state ☐
Phobic state ☐
Obsessive compulsive disorder ☐
Other (specify) ☐

3. MENTAL HEALTH THREAT - FURTHER ISSUES

a) Is it a problem which is organically or psychosocially caused?
b) Is it a problem which can be resolved without medication?
c) If medication is required, what are the likely consequences of failing to take medication?
d) Is further deterioration likely regardless of need for medication?
e) Does the problem appear stable and difficult to shift?

---

*Note that *dependence* on alcohol or drugs alone does not fall within the ambit of the Act, in terms of its definition of mental disorder (Section 1).

Comments:

4. MENTAL HEALTH THREAT: SUPPLEMENTARY FACTORS

Requires medication to resolve ☐
Deterioration without medication ☐
Permanent mental health consequences without medication ☐
Social circumstances fraught ☐
Stable mental health condition with deteriorating social functioning ☐

5. SEVERITY RATING   SIGNIFICANCE RATING
   (MENTAL HEALTH)   (SUPPLEMENTARY FACTORS)

Very severe	☐	5	Very significant	☐	5
Quite severe	☐	4	Quite significant	☐	4
Moderate	☐	3	Moderate	☐	3
Mild to moderate	☐	2	Mild to moderate	☐	2
Mild	☐	1	Mild	☐	1
Not present	☐	0	Not present	☐	0

CLASSIFICATION 3: PHYSICAL ILL HEALTH THREAT

1. BROAD ILL HEALTH THREAT CLASSIFICATION:
Indicate which of the following represents the ill health threat.

a. Life threatening ☐
b. Threatening permanent disability ☐
c. Requiring specialist hospital treatment ☐
d. Requiring specialist out-patient treatment ☐
e. Requiring treatment by GP ☐
f. Self-limiting or transient ☐
g. No physical illness ☐

2. PHYSICAL ILL HEALTH: VULNERABILITIES:
Do any of the following exist which may exacerbate the physical ill health threat?

Age related (elderly) frailty ☐
Already frail but not elderly ☐
Already suffering physical ill health ☐
Already weakened (e.g. exhausted by hyperactivity or sleeplessness) ☐
Environmental vulnerability ☐
(e.g. homelessness/inadequate housing etc.)

3. SEVERITY RATING (PHYSICAL ILL HEALTH)

Very severe ☐ 5
Quite severe ☐ 4
Moderate ☐ 3
Mild to moderate ☐ 2
Mild ☐ 1
Not present ☐ 0

SIGNIFICANCE RATING (VULNERABILITY)

Very significant ☐ 5
Quite significant ☐ 4
Moderate ☐ 3
Mild to moderate ☐ 2
Mild ☐ 1
Not present ☐ 0

CLASSIFICATION 4: SAFETY THREAT

Indicate if the patient is threatened with the loss of any of the following (column A)

Indicate if the patient is vulnerable in any threatened loss area (column B)

	A	B
Life (i.e. threat of death)	☐	☐
Physical integrity (injury threat)	☐	☐
Sexual integrity (threat of rape/sex assault/exploitation)	☐	☐
Family	☐	☐
Spouse	☐	☐

SEE OVER

	A	B
Child(ren)	☐	☐
Social relationships	☐	☐
Employment	☐	☐
Finances	☐	☐
Other material goods	☐	☐
Non-offender status (threat of arrest/prosecution)	☐	☐
Other (specify)	☐	☐

Describe briefly the vulnerabilities that the patient has in those areas where their safety is threatened (e.g. if loss of spouse is threatened are there any vulnerabilities in this area?)

SEVERITY RATING
(SAFETY THREAT)

Very severe	☐	5
Quite severe	☐	4
Moderate	☐	3
Mild to moderate	☐	2
Mild	☐	1

SIGNIFICANCE RATING
(VULNERABILITY)

Very significant	☐	5
Quite significant	☐	4
Moderate	☐	3
Mild to moderate	☐	2
Mild	☐	1

CLASSIFICATION 5: PROTECTION OF OTHER PERSONS

1. PROTECTION REQUIRED FROM:

Death ☐
Physical harm/injury ☐

SEE OVER

Physical ill health ☐
Mental ill health ☐
Sub-mental health emotional trauma ☐
Children's stability/disruption of emotional development ☐
Family separation ☐
Reputation/personal integrity (libel) ☐
Intrusive behaviour (pestering people/creating a disturbance/shouting/banging walls ☐
Offending public taste (publicly swearing/public nakedness etc.) ☐
Other (specify) ☐

2. FOCUS (who requires protection)

Husband/male cohabitee	☐	Other female relatives	☐
Wife/female cohabitee	☐	Neighbours	☐
Male friend/boyfriend	☐	Acquaintances (not neighbours)	☐
Female friend/girlfriend	☐	Officials & professionals	☐
Child	☐	Work colleagues	☐
Elderly person	☐	'Generalised others'	☐
Other male relatives	☐	Other (specify)	☐

3. Describe briefly any vulnerabilities others have (if any) in those areas where they require protection.

4. SEVERITY RATING   SIGNIFICANCE RATING
   (OTHERS' PROTECTION)   (VULNERABILITY)

Very severe	☐ 5	Very significant	☐ 5
Quite severe	☐ 4	Quite significant	☐ 4
Moderate	☐ 3	Moderate	☐ 3
Mild to moderate	☐ 2	Mild to moderate	☐ 2
Mild	☐ 1	Mild	☐ 1
Not present	☐ 0	Not present	☐ 0

SERIOUSNESS OF DANGER - OVERALL RATING

Very serious	☐
Quite serious	☐
Moderate	☐
Mild to moderate	☐
Mild	☐
Not present	☐

LEVEL OF RISK

BEHAVIOUR OF THE PATIENT: ITS CONTRIBUTION TO THE LIKELIHOOD OF DANGER OCCURRING

a) Is the behaviour of the patient contributing to the increased probability of danger?
b) If so, how likely are they to change their behaviour as the danger becomes more manifest?
c) Is the danger itself transitory or self-limiting?
d) Is the patient sufficiently in control of themselves to prevent the danger occurring?

CLASSIFICATION 6: AVAILABILITY AND ADEQUACY OF SUPPORT

a) What support is *required* to maintain the patient in the community?
b) Is that support *available?*

c) Is the support available from support provider *adequate?* In particular:
   1. What capacity does the support provider have to provide sufficient support to reduce the level of risk to an acceptable level?
   2. Will the support provider be able to sustain the support for a sufficiently long time?

	SUPPORT		
	Required	Available	Adequate
INSTRUMENTAL:			
Food/cooking	☐	☐	☐
Accommodation	☐	☐	☐
Nursing/health supervision	☐	☐	☐
Personal physical aid (e.g. lifting patient)	☐	☐	☐
Supervision of eating	☐	☐	☐
Supervision of finances (e.g. DSS benefits/payment of bills)	☐	☐	☐
Supervision of taking medication	☐	☐	☐
Home management/cleaning/shopping	☐	☐	☐
Physical supervision of children	☐	☐	☐
Physical supervision of other dependents	☐	☐	☐
Personal hygiene supervision	☐	☐	☐
Monitoring behaviour (e.g. to prevent overdose)	☐	☐	☐
Other (specify)	☐	☐	☐
PSYCHOLOGICAL:			
Emotional support/ventilation	☐	☐	☐
Psychodynamic support (cognitive and to resolve emotional problems)	☐	☐	☐
Emotional support for patient's distressed dependents	☐	☐	☐
Providing children's emotional/developmental needs (e.g. stable emotionally significant relative)	☐	☐	☐
Other (specify)	☐	☐	☐

SUPPORT PROVIDER(S) AVAILABLE: include statement of why they are considered adequate.

a) *Formal:* (e.g. nurse, social worker, home help, voluntary worker etc.)

b) *Informal:* (e.g. spouse, other relative, neighbour, landlord/lady, friend/acquaintance)

COLLECTION OF INFORMATION: THOSE INTERVIEWED AS PART OF THE ASSESSMENT PROCESS.

a) Were the main relevant individuals interviewed as part of the assessment process? Who were those people interviewed?

b) Where some relevant individuals were not interviewed, why was this?

LEVEL OF RISK:	High Risk	☐
	Fairly High Risk	☐
	Moderate Risk	☐
	Fairly Low Risk	☐
	Low Risk	☐

OVERALL RATING OF RISK (OVERALL RISK)

Level of Risk:

Seriousness of Danger:

PART FOUR

THE ROLE OF THE ASW IN CONTEXT

The special importance of compulsory admissions for social work practice lies in its combination of professional issues and civil rights. The professional issues are complex, since there is a combination of factors which makes the ASW unique in social work: when undertaking assessment for compulsory admissions he is acting as an independent professional in his own right rather than as an agency representative; he is expected, by law, to possess 'appropriate competence' and not to act 'in bad faith' or 'without reasonable care'; he is working in an environment independent of the courts where he is legally required to co-operate with a separate profession - medicine - in order to section a patient; and the field in which he works is *defined* as mental health rather than social work (hence the Mental Health Act). Yet the civil rights issues are of equal importance: the ASW confronts situations (at times) where the courts would not have grounds to imprison an individual, yet they have the right - with doctors - to deprive them of their freedom by hospitalising them; they are expected to operate with cognitive superiority - their expertise means that their (combined with doctors') definition of the situation rather than that of the client is all important; and this happens without reference to the courts or justices of the peace. Notwithstanding all this, the ASWs operate within the 'open texture' of the law in which they do not possess the guidance of precedent or case law. The ASW is, therefore, in a position of extreme responsibility and possesses great power.

Yet if anything comes over from the research it is the potential breadth of possible interpretations of the 'health or safety of the patient' and 'protection of others' criteria, together with the opportunity for inconsistencies in interpretation between different ASWs. In retrospect this is hardly surprising: social work, like any profession, contains diverse groups of people, with differing beliefs and commitments and, notwithstanding the unifying effects of professional socialisation (Pavalko, 1971), differences in behaviour are perhaps inevitable. However, if we find differences exist within a single team, with the possible unifying effect of both frequent contact and the likelihood that they will, as many social workers do (Stevenson and Parsloe, 1978), discuss their cases, how great will the variations be in different teams up and down the country?

Indeed, we may have been forewarned by the experience of psychiatrists in the process of diagnosis. Clare (1980) states that:

> 'There is disquieting evidence that suggests that under ordinary clinical conditions psychiatric diagnosis can be extremely unreliable.'

He points to a number of significant studies showing considerable differences between psychiatrists even working in the same hospital in their diagnosis of patients. One study (Passamanick et al, 1959) concluded that:

> 'Despite protestations that their point of reference is always the individual patient, clinicians may in fact be so committed to a particular psychiatric diagnosis that the patient's treatment is largely predetermined.'

Echoes here of the impact of the mental health orientation, discussed earlier, on section assessments. Perhaps the lesson to be learned is that we cannot hope to achieve complete consistency, but that we can strive for improvements. This lesson should be applied to health or safety of the patient and protection of others criteria.

The development of a social risk *orientation,* however, can be related to the assessment schedule learning process. Its primary purpose is, of course, the development of relevant knowledge and skills. Its secondary *effect,* however, can be the related socialisation process. Pavalko (1971) calls this the means by which people:

> 'take on the characteristics of their culture - its values, beliefs and assumptions about what are and are not appropriate ways of behaving through the process of learning'.

The outcome of socialisation is to produce conformity to shared values, norms and expectations about role behaviour. Certainly in-depth focussed examination of the analysis of the process of assessment of health or safety of patients and protection of others provides a forum, particularly in ASW training, through which shared expectations may be developed.

However, this form of post-qualification occupational socialisation carries with it certain provisos. Adult socialisation involves, in addition to learning new roles and norms, the unlearning and relinquishing of old norms and roles, as well as the extension of old roles. Additionally, unlike children undergoing socialisation, the adult is relatively free to escape from socialising experiences considered intolerable or distasteful. These factors are particularly important when entering an occupation: a person entering social work training may have come with certain expectations and may become disillusioned if these expectations are not realised and as a result leave the profession. This is far more unlikely with ASW training: as a post-qualification training the social workers have already been subject to the socialisation processes involved in taking on an occupational identity, and will additionally have a clearer idea about the ASW training and role before embarking on them.

Furthermore, various socialisation mechanisms function to exert control over the behaviour of individual practitioners and encourage uniformity in expectations and values. The occupation becomes a major normative reference group whose norms, values and definitions of appropriate occupational conduct serve as guides by which the individual practitioner organises and performs his own work. This may occur, for example, through formal channels, such as codes of ethics. Informal channels involve, for example, positive personal evaluations by their colleagues. To the extent that individuals are strongly identified with their occupation group, the seeking of colleague approval gives colleagues a high degree of control over the individual's behaviour and legitimates efforts to socialise him further.

Certainly, therefore, a growing concern with the area of the health or safety of the patient and protection of others, a greater clarity when analysing it, and an increasing sensitisation to civil rights issues may be seen as much an aspect of socialisation as education, which would accompany an increased and detailed focus in this area.

The Social Work Element of Compulsory Admissions

The role of ASWs in compulsory admission assessments has been conceptualised as that of gatekeeper. The concept of the ASW as gatekeeper goes a considerable way to identifying how the roles of ASW and medical practitioner differ, thus giving the ASW a distinctive and highly significant identity in the assessment process. The key to this is a reconceptualising of the mental health problem as a social problem. This is not an anti-psychiatric stance; indeed it would not be consistent with the *Mental Health* Act for this to be the case. Instead, it is necessary to carry this definition alongside that of mental health, so that they operate in parallel. This can be taken as a metaphor for the way in which, ideally, doctors and ASWs may operate alongside each other in practice. In taking this line the ASW role is related to the social work task while also defining mental health issues socially.

David Howe (1979) has identified two critical dimensions of social work practice: that it is carried out under 'social auspices' and involves matters of 'social concern'. This is a definition of social work as function and it means, essentially, that social work can only be carried out where authorised by an appropriate social authority - the state - and that it involves matters about which social concern is expressed, which are perceived as social problems. This, he argues, is expressed through agency function, and the social worker's authority rests ultimately on his relationship to his agency. For the ASW matters are slightly different: the agency is largely given its function through statute, hence it acts as an intermediary between the law and the practitioners. In the case of compulsory admissions, the ASW acts as an independent professional, and hence has a more direct relationship with the law which empowers him.

A further dimension of this involves reconceptualising psychiatric symptoms as residual rule-breaking, without in other respects committing ourselves to a labelling perspective explaining mental illness entirely as the result of a 'social reaction'. Residual rule-breaking places the patient in his social context: that the behaviour which is causing social concern is the result of rarely considered assumptions about what constitutes 'acceptable' or 'normal' behaviour, and which make the patient's behaviour incomprehensible. In this way it is clear that the puzzlement about the behaviour of a patient arises in a group or social context where perceptions of behaviour are governed by norms. This may be stated while remaining quite agnostic about the *cause* of the particular problems, which may be biological, social or psychological. However, it clearly indicates how it is a matter of social concern, a concern which has been enshrined in statute.

This perhaps partly explains the Mental Health Act Commission's desire to see, where necessary, patients compulsorily admitted for mental ill health alone. For if their behaviour is residual rule-breaking, then it may be both incomprehensible and a matter of concern. It is perhaps not surprising if this concern is expressed in a way that includes mental health under the criteria of 'health or safety' of the patient.

The issues can be seen as 'social' in further ways. There is now extensive evidence of the impact of social factors on mental illness. Social factors, in this context, refer to the influence, direct or indirect, of social structures or institutions, on the individuals or groups concerned (Boskoff, 1971).

Thus adverse social conditions, poor housing, unemployment, poverty and so on, are related to a raised incidence of mental illness (Cochrane, 1983). Life events and longer term difficulties are identified as causal factors in some disorders such as depressions (Brown and Harris, 1978), while life events can precipitate schizophrenia, an illness with a strong genetic component (Brown and Birley, 1968). Likewise social supports are perceived either to provide a buffer (or protection) against mental illness, in the face of adverse provoking factors, or their absence is seen as a causal factor in mental illness (Henderson, 1984). Indeed, these and other factors have been combined to form a social causal model of depression (Brown and Harris, 1978; Brown et al, 1987; Brown, 1987). Furthermore, social factors in the form of the patient's environment may influence prognosis for both neurotic and psychotic patients (Weissman and Paykel, 1974). Finally, the mentally ill person may have a seriously burdening effect on their carers, thus affecting their capacity to care adequately for him (Miles, 1987). Thus social factors relate to cause, process and prognosis of mental illness.

These social factors give the ASW a formidable claim to their role. It is quite different from the claim of the medical practitioner which rests primarily on their definition of the problem in terms of health, and their expertise in this area. For them, then, the social considerations take second place to health in their claim, while for ASWs the reverse is the case. This analysis, additionally, throws further light on whether the ASW role could be taken on by the community psychiatric nurse (CPN). It could not, because the *nature* of the CPN role and social work differs. ASWs are concerned with mental health and compulsory admissions primarily as a social problem - hence it is carried out under social auspices with matters of social concern. Their role in compulsory admissions is entirely consistent with their role in other areas, and reflects the very nature of social work.

The ASW Role and Use of Assessment Schedule

The assessment schedule has been developed in recognition of the 'open texture' of the relevant law, and because it may contribute to the development of expertise among ASWs. It is consistent with the social risk orientation advocated here for ASWs and, by providing a 'knowledge base', may contribute to the development of this orientation in the face of detailed diagnostic criteria and knowledge available on mental health. Most critically, in terms of our analysis of the role of the ASW, its use, by providing a knowledge base for assessment, has a major effect on the *way* the role is carried out.

Within these broad aims, the schedule's primary objective is to help clarify the assessment process and secondly to provide for a reduced threshold of risk. Certainly greater clarity of analysis may well reduce the threshold of risk simply because the ASW will thereby be more precise about the likely consequences of failure to admit, thus inconsistencies would be less likely to arise from obfuscation on the part of the ASW. Further reduction in the threshold of risk requires ASWs as a whole to interpret the law with a similar degree of breadth or narrowness, or to have it more precisely defined for them by precedent or statute. It may be that the development of a knowledge base for analysing the health or safety of the patient or protection of others, together with a social risk orientation, will contribute to this process by focussing specifically on these criteria, uncluttered by the related but separate assessment of mental disorder.

How helpful, however, is the development of the assessment schedule in the provision of a knowledge base for social work in this area? The approach adopted here is an example of 'practice-led' research, which may be contrasted with 'theory-driven' practice. 'Practice-led' research entails that the approach is consistent with the nature and limits of social work. Thus the research focusses on a particular problem - compulsory mental health admissions - and its related issues of practice law, civil rights and knowledge. However, it *also* adopts assumptions consistent with the nature of social work which, as Davies (1985) points out, are essentially consensus and functionalist. The outcome is research which is useful to practice because it adopts the same frame of reference as that of social work. This does not mean it is not evaluative, or is uncritical - indeed this research is both evaluative and critical. It does mean, however, that recommendations may be made which, because they fit with the framework of practice, are realistic and possible to adopt by social work. It is no coincidence that the assessment schedule was, to a considerable extent, *generated* by the research. For social work, research is not an end in itself but is a facilitator of practice: an urgency is added by the need to 'do something' about problems, and the objectives of academics are only the servant or facilitator of this aim (Sheppard, 1984). Thus the twin principles of 'practice-led' research are *specificity* - that the research should concentrate specifically on particular problems and issues of social work - and *congruence* - that the frame of reference of both research and practice should be similar.

This may be contrasted with 'theory-driven' practice. Here the recommendations for practice are not based on an understanding of the nature of social work, but on an image of social work derived from theory. For example, Corrigan and Leonard (1978), on the basis of their theory, created an image of social workers as political revolutionaries with no more than a fleeting resemblance to *actual practice.* Unrestrained by the discipline of a focus and framework derived from practice, the social worker, in Corrigan and Leonard's world, was free to change the very nature of society. The social work role, regardless of real life circumstances, was essentially derived from theory. Of course this was fantasy, the more so in view of subsequent political developments.

Although a stark example, the principle holds true for all 'theory-led' images of practice. The sociologist cannot determine the nature of social work practice, but 'practice-led' social research can be very useful. This does not mean 'practice-led' research is atheoretical, as this study I hope demonstrates, but that only theoretical perspectives consistent with the assumptions of social work practice can generate research useful to practice.

Furthermore, congruence and specificity move us away from old style 'general theories' of social work, such as psychosocial, existentialist or marxist, as the *way forward* for social work. By their very generality they do not provide social workers with specific guides to specific problems, and are conflicting and contradictory. 'Practice-led' research, more modest and piecemeal, involves detailed research carried out on particular problems and issues, within a theoretical framework consistent with social work assumptions.

Many of the principles underlying the development of the assessment schedule were discussed at the beginning of the Part Three. However, its distinctiveness from two other approaches should be identified. First, it should not be mistaken for a checklist, examples of which have been developed in particular in relation to the detection of child abuse (White-Franklin, 1977). Although based on research - some of which, however, is dubious (Sheppard, 1982) - these are essentially unidimensional. They simply present a list of possible 'risk factors' which, while they direct the social worker to particular areas, are ticked or not according to their presence or absence.

Our assessment schedule is multi-dimensional, and operates on a number of conceptually distinct levels. The first involves the classification of broad domains of hazard, danger, risk and evidence. Within these, at a second level, lie further classifications in the form of categories generated within their domains, or as questions which relate to that particular domain. These factors are examined in terms of vulnerability and protective factors which increase or reduce the risk to the patient. Finally, these factors are examined in order to evaluate the overall risk to the patient, eventually based on the seriousness of the danger and level of risk. It is arguable, therefore, that it provides a considerably more sophisticated knowledge base than a checklist.

Goldberg and Huxley (1980) have commented that:

> 'The social work role in relation to the mentally ill client has in most local authorities become stagnant, and the emphasis has remained upon outdated methods of intervention which has led to the atrophy of skill development.'

They point to the poverty of theory-based work arising from the marginalising of the mentally ill as a group. This contrasts with clinical psychology whose:

> 'Techniques are of proven value (while)...social workers lack a sufficiently coherent theoretical underpinning.'

To some degree developments since Goldberg and Huxley wrote, particularly ASW training, have created a greater awareness of mental health issues in this specialist group. In some areas, such as task-centred work, social work does possess a coherent and usable theoretical base. However, it is Kate Woof's research which demonstrates most clearly the significance of social work training in practice (Woof, 1987). She compared mental health social workers with community psychiatric nurses in their management of psychiatric patients. Although her findings are complex, the major elements in relation to social workers were that they used their considerable counselling and casework skills extensively, were able to mobilise various welfare facilities, and initiated and maintained clients' links with non-health agencies. The community psychiatric nurses, by contrast, provided long-term monitoring and administration of medication for schizophrenic clients, and were able to listen with understanding to clients' problems and provide reassurance, advice and support. While clearly in some respects the strengths of these occupations lay in different areas, Woof commented that the nurses were able to offer only 'simple psychotherapy' - emotional support - compared to the far more advanced counselling and problem solving skills (psychotherapy) offered by the social workers, while the latter were more effective in the use of welfare facilities and provision of links with non-health agencies. This, Woof considered, was primarily the product of training, and it is easy to recognise - when social workers are not suffering any crisis of confidence - that these rest on theory-based occupational skills developed in social work which have simply been applied to clients with mental health problems.

Woof's research indicates, in the realm of psychiatry, that the knowledge and skills base of an occupation has an impact on the ways its practitioners work and hence the way they carry out their role. The development of the assessment schedule, with its concomitant development and application of concepts and issues for the purpose of more systematic assessment, represents a further 'theoretical underpinning' for mental health social work which will help prevent 'outdated methods of intervention' and the 'atrophy of skill development'.

Mental Health and Social Functioning

The issue of including mental health as an aspect of 'health or safety of the patient' remains a tantalising one despite this research. The ASW is not greatly helped by the comments of the Mental Health Act Commission in this respect: in view of the confusion it is not surprising that some patients are sectioned for mental illness alone, while in other cases further risk factors in addition to mental illness are required to admit them compulsorily. It is interesting that only psychotic patients were admitted for reasons of mental health alone. However, other patients showing psychotic symptoms were neither compulsorily nor informally admitted, even where the ASW felt in principle that they would benefit from treatment. Clearly, compulsory admission for these patients was seen as an infringement of their civil rights.

The presence of psychosis, therefore, was not alone sufficient to account for these admissions. A further concept is required; that of social functioning appears particularly helpful in this respect. Without clearly identifying social functioning as an issue, the ASWs in some of the relevant cases (although not all) displayed a dim awareness of its significance. Thus, one ASW commented of a patient in his own inimitable way that:

> 'Her mental health was very poor. Judging from previous reports she was a together lady, quite able to manage her finances, home, life and so on.'

Another ASW sectioned a man because:

> 'He was deluded with religious ideas. He had seen visions of the end of the world. He was *totally out of touch with reality.*' (my italics)

Both these accounts appeal to some notion of social functioning. Social functioning, or social adjustment, is a concept well understood in psychiatry as it is seen to be frequently deleteriously affected by mental illness. However, and this is highly significant for the ASW role, social functioning has been put forward as a concept which distinguishes social work from other activities (Bartlett, 1970).

Platt (1981) conducted a useful study of the concept of social adjustment used by psychiatrists. Although highly critical of their measures he presents the central elements of the concept. It is founded, he says, 'on the interrelation between the individual and his environment' and he uses role analysis as a framework for examining this relationship. Platt draws on sociological work to expand this further. He sees role as 'a set of evaluative standards applied to an incumbent of a particular position': it involves a set of expectations of what is involved in that role and how well it should be carried out. Hence the role of father may involve emotional nurturing, disciplining, protecting the child, breadwinning and so on. However, the role is carried out in a specific social location, which introduces the concept of 'role set'. This is the complement of role relations which persons have by virtue of occupying a particular social status. For example, the school teacher has a distinctive role set relating the teacher to pupils, colleagues, the school head, professional teacher organisations and so on. This constitutes their 'social location'.

However, 'social location' has two further implications. The first is the variability of role expectations, i.e. what a person should do in order to fulfil the particular role. Expectations of a particular role may be 'heterogeneous and often conflicting' according to the particular audience concerned: there is not a single uniform set of cultural expectations associated with a particular position. Social workers may, amongst some groups, be seen to be in the business of separating children and families; to others they aim to *prevent* separation.

Second, role *performance* is subject to variable expectations: this is the actual conduct expected of an individual while on duty in his position. To evaluate the performance of roles, it is necessary to take account of the expectations that are current in the person's own social group. Both role expectations and role performance arise because of segmentation in society, with its various subcultures, involving different standards derived from reference groups.

Bartlett (1970) developed the closely related concept of social functioning to identify the *focus* for social work, rather in the way that health and illness provide the focus for medical intervention. Bartlett sees the focus of social work to be the 'interaction between people and environment' which leads to social functioning or dysfunctioning. She states that this interaction between person and environment is a consistent theme in social work literature. Social functioning involves related concepts.

1. Tasks: these are activities which people fulfil in their performance of particular roles. They are concerned with the situation to be dealt with by the client.

2. Coping: having described the nature of life tasks, the next issue is how people actually deal with these tasks. If they are able to perform these tasks they are said to be coping: if they are not, they are not coping. Coping is the 'relative mastery of the tasks involved in the situation'.

3. Environmental demands: failure to master a task may be the result of failings or difficulties in the person themselves. However it may also, or alternatively, be the result of the environment: many will suffer stress in dealing with life tasks, but some 'will be able to take the necessary steps without becoming disturbed or disorganised'. Others, who fail, may do so because the 'demands of the environment' are excessive in relation to the coping capacity of the people involved in the situation. Poverty, racial discrimination, lack of access to jobs and so on, 'subject large segments of the population to stress, anxiety, deprivation and alienation'.

The social worker is left with the questions, 'Are the environmental demands excessive?' and 'Are people's coping capacities inadequate?'. If there is an imbalance, further, how can the balance be improved?

The concept of social functioning, then, involves the interaction of people with their environment in a form of 'exchange balance'. In helping people to deal with their life situations, Bartlett thinks, the social worker must understand the *meaning* of the situations to the people involved in them; this does not refer simply to the client, but to others who are jointly affected by the situation or who are affected by the client's task performance. This concept is closely allied to 'social adjustment'. It involves the interrelation between the individual and the environment; it involves role performance, closely related to coping; and it places this in its subcultural context by identifying the meaning of the situation for the participants.

The concepts of social functioning and social adjustment have potential when considering admissions on mental health grounds alone. The Mental Health Act Commission (1987) states that:

'Sections 2 and 3 both allow for detention on the grounds of the patient's health (including mental health).....if the patient's condition deteriorates.'

They appear to suggest that the deterioration concerned is health deterioration, which is not, it appears, social functioning. However, in the case of mental health, deterioration may be most apparent when *indicated* by increasing problems with social functioning. In practice situations ASWs may well ask themselves: this person is depressed (or anxious or psychotic) but can they manage adequately in the community? If the answer is 'yes' (and there are no other health or safety of the patient or protection of others risks) the ASW is quite likely not to admit the patient compulsorily. This would go a long way to explaining why a number of patients with psychotic symptoms were not admitted.

Of course the Act does not allow admission on the grounds of social maladjustment or social dysfunctioning of mentally disordered people. There appear two possible ways forward. First, if social dysfunctioning were taken as an indication of the seriousness of the mental health problem, this would fit with the criteria. However, for this to be the case, social dysfunctioning would have to be viewed as an aspect of mental disorder (i.e. a defining element) rather than a *consequence* of mental disorder (i.e. closely related but separate). Furthermore, it would be consistent with our approach only if this rule was made explicit and some indication of the factors to be examined was provided. The importance of guidance to assist clarity in assessment has already been demonstrated. This might most easily be given through the Memorandum of the Biennial Report of the Mental Health Act Commission.

The second alternative involves adding social dysfunctioning to the criteria of the health or safety of the patient or the protection of other persons. This would mean that no-one would be sectioned on the grounds of mental ill health alone, but additionally it would take place with a view to the health or safety *or* social functioning of the patient (or the protection of other persons). This approach denies the possibility of subsuming social functioning under the broad domain of health. This does not mean that mental illness does not affect social functioning. Impairment of role performance related, for example, to child care or employment may well occur in the face of mental disorder. The argument that it is conceptually distinct is based, however, on the fact that impaired role performance may occur *without* the presence of mental illness. Hence, the person performing badly in their work may do so because of poor relations with their colleagues, boredom, disillusionment with the ethics of the work they do, and so on. If this approach was taken it would be insufficient for the Mental Health Act Commission to give advice on the interpretation of the Act (since social functioning would not be an aspect of health) but would require amendment to the Act. Whichever of these two alternatives is adopted the analysis of the component elements suggests certain factors to be examined:

1. The ASW needs to know *which roles* are significant to assess, e.g. employment, parental, home care etc.

2. The ASW needs to evaluate the role in relation to *subcultural expectations*. What is expected of this person in their role in their particular circumstances (middle class, working class, black, white, female, male and so on)?

3. The ASW needs to identify what constitutes *adequate role performance* of the particular tasks or expectations attached to the role.

4. To achieve this, as Platt suggests, the ASW should 'take into account the views of the subject's significant others in arriving at both a description and an evaluation of role performance'.

However, this is not simply a matter of practice assessment. Drawing upon social functioning is important in terms of the nature of the ASW role. Social functioning - or social adjustment - may be of interest to the psychiatrist because it is affected by mental illness. However, according to Bartlett it is a *defining characteristic* of social work as it constitutes the *focus for* social work, rather as health and illness provide the focus for medicine. If social functioning represents a significant factor in compulsory admission on mental health grounds alone, this provides further evidence of the central and distinctive role for social work inherent in the Mental Health Act. It is, so to speak, social work terrain.

However, our conceptual schema does not allow the incorporation of social functioning as a social work element of the Act without reference to further factors. It has previously been shown how, in Howe's words, social work is carried out under 'social auspices' with matters of 'social concern'. Hence it is carried out primarily in duly authorised agencies on matters of social concern such as child abuse, mental illness, mental handicap/learning difficulties and so on. Where does social functioning fit into this? Social workers are not, for example, to be seen rushing around after tramps, or with all aspects of homelessness where this is affecting a person's ability to sustain employment or social relationships. Hence social workers are not always involved with all aspects of social functioning; their work is delimited in some way. Social functioning should be seen as a secondary *practice focus* for social work: it is secondary to the primary *territorial focus* on issues of social concern which are carried out under social auspices. Thus, the social worker will be concerned with the potentially child abusing parent, and will focus on their social functioning - in particular their ability to carry out their child care role. In so doing they may work on a variety of factors, environmental and personal, to reduce the risk of child abuse. The position of the ASW described here is exactly the same: their involvement with mental health, and compulsory admissions in particular, arises because these are issues of social concern; their work is carried out under social auspices - the law; and in relation to our suggestion about compulsory admissions the practice focus is on the patient's social functioning.

Social Conflict - Medical Collaboration: Creative Tension or Conflict?

A major objective of the 1983 Act was to improve the standing of the social workers acting in compulsory admission cases in the eyes of other professionals. The training required for appropriate competence, and the powers and the duties under the Act, both contributed to this although ASWs may still be bypassed by the nearest relative if they refuse to apply for hospital admission. The ASW role is to act independently of, rather than subordinate to, the medical role.

However, as a result of their increased status and independence, as Anderson-Ford and Hasley (1984) point out:

> 'The possibility of conflict between doctors and approved social workers is built into the Act. In theory, the roles appear quite separate. In practice, however, there is substantial overlap in the roles of the doctor and approved social worker, and it is in this area that disputes can occur.'

Thus, for example, the ASW must indicate in relation to Section 3 that hospital detention is the 'most appropriate' way of providing care and treatment, while the medical recommendation must indicate that it is 'appropriate' that the patient receives treatment in hospital which cannot be provided without Section 3 detention. Conflict might arise if the ASW feels treatment may be provided in a less restrictive environment and the doctor(s) does not.

However, there is a different *emphasis* in the ASW and medical role (Anderson-Ford and Hasley, 1984).

'The doctor examines the patient, makes a medical diagnosis, and completes an appropriate medical recommendation, whilst the approved social worker decides on *social work principles* whether or not the patient should be admitted to hospital.' (my italics)

This, indeed, is the rub, for the principles underlying social work, and those underlying medicine, do not always coincide as was illustrated earlier in relation to 'respect for persons' (social work) and 'respect for life' (medicine). This reflects differences in the 'assumptive worlds' of the two occupations - arising from commonly held approaches, assumptions, attitudes and standards *within* the occupation, which are however different from those of other occupations (Pavalko, 1971; Huntington, 1981). We have already shown that the status and role of the ASW is quite different from that of the medical practitioner - conceptualising the ASW as a rule-enforcing gatekeeper, concerned with mental health because of its status as a social problem, acting under social auspices in a matter of social concern. Additionally illness, whether physical or mental, is normative and hence has a social dimension which links mental health to social concerns. The ASW has an incorrigibly social role, and although he is expected to utilise mental health knowledge, possesses a knowledge base primarily derived from the social sciences. Doctors' involvement derives from their professional claim to 'own' the territory concerned: health, including mental health, is 'their' area and their status derives from their expertise in diagnosis and treatment.

This is reflected in the 'assumptive world' of the doctor. The greatest imperative in medicine, as enshrined in the Hippocratic Oath, is the preservation of life and treatment of the sick. In Bean's (1980) study of the 1959 Act, this emerged in the form of what he called therapeutic particularism. This meant that exclusive attention was directed towards the individual patient and that the major interest was for the patient's health or welfare. When clashes occurred between the requirements of the legal rules and the requirements of the patient's welfare, the latter was regarded as the most important. The psychiatrists often engaged in *ad hoc* balancing of interests which resisted reduction to general rules. As a result some patients were admitted illegally, while others were admitted under the 'emergency' Section (29) when a second doctor could have been obtained.

The mental health orientation, with its emphasis on the mental health status of the patient, entails less concentration on the detailed analysis of factors related to health of the patient or protection of others. Although different from therapeutic particularism, it also has its roots in the treatment needs of the patient. The basic requirement to treat the sick, plus the existence of therapeutic particularism, provides philosophical and circumstantial evidence that a mental health orientation is predominant in medicine. This is further emphasised in the research by the overall lack of differences between ASWs and doctors in their assessments.

There are, furthermore, wider issues relating to medicine and social work as a whole which have been identified by Huntington (1981) for which compulsory admission assessments may provide a focus. One issue relates to individual (clinical) versus collective (environmental) orientations. Doctors concentrate normally on the health or sickness of individual patients while social workers lay emphasis on relationships within the family, community and society as a whole. Not only do they possess a different focus but:

> 'because of this difference in orientation, the concepts used by each occupation tend also to be different, so that communication within some common frame of reference may be difficult to achieve' (Huntington, 1981).

Social work training alerts social workers to environmental factors in a way not available with medical training (although it should be said that psychiatrists have shown a greater concern as a whole with 'social' factors than most of their medical colleagues). Indeed, 'environmental factors' have been explicitly included in the assessment schedule (see above) through which the ASW would be expected to identify, for example, vulnerabilities in the patient's situation and the availability and adequacy of social supports. A more comprehensive analysis of these factors may lead to conclusions about the level of risk and seriousness of danger which are different from judgements derived *solely* from considering the patient themselves. Potential differences occur, therefore, not simply because of the individual versus collective foci of medicine and social work, but because these are channelled through the use of the assessment schedule which analyses the health or safety of the patient or protection of others.

A further element, mentioned previously, is the 'action' orientation of medicine contrasting with the 'holding' orientation of social work. The doctors predilection for 'doing' must be related back to training, in which the dominant image of the emergency prevails. Either the doctor acts or the patient dies. Social work, by contrast, emphasises the importance of carefully thought-out alternatives, which can take time. Both social work education and practice teach that precipitate and ill thought-out action can be disastrous. Alongside this exist the emotions of the individuals involved: a person socialised to take action, and behave as if circumstances are emergencies even when they are not, is liable to feel a high level of anxiety if some kind of action is not taken. Social workers though are expected to live with risk throughout their professional lives, because neither the law nor their knowledge base (nor perhaps their physical powers) give them control over their areas of responsibility which would allow that risk to be reduced. Most social workers, for example, have potential child abuse cases where for a variety of reasons a child must remain in a 'risky' environment. When a situation lies within the domain of health, as with mental health sections, and it has all the *appearances* of an emergency (as indeed compulsory admissions sometimes are), the individual with an action orientation is not only likely to feel anxious, but feel *justified* in their anxiety, even when time is available to explore alternatives and make a more considered decision. Again the use of the assessment schedule, emphasising the development of a considered decision, taking time where practical, provides a focus for this aspect of social work.

A final element of relevance here is the presumption of medical dominance. Huntington points out that while articles about 'teams' written by non-medical authors are general replete with democratic imagery this is not the case with general practitioners. They are perceived as the 'spiders' at the centre of a web of services, while other team members are seen as their surrogates. Ultimate responsibility rests with the GP; he must therefore be 'captain of his ship'.

What is true of general practice is doubly true of hospital specialists. Consultants are perceived to be at the pinnacle of medicine, and have a status above that of general practitioners. This is true of consultant psychiatrists, even though they are lower in the status hierarchy than other medical specialists such as surgeons. Indeed, Bean's (1980) research showed the extent to which general practitioners were led by the psychiatrists when assessing compulsory admissions.

However, the ASW, when considering sectioning a patient, is not working *in* a team, headed by a doctor or doctors, but working *with* these doctors. Their role is deliberately designed to give them independence from, rather than subordination to, the medical practitioners involved and they possess specific rights and duties in this respect. However, independence from doctors provides the opportunity also to come to different decisions, particularly as the ASW is expected to possess 'appropriate competence'. This may not be appreciated by doctors for various reasons. First, an assumption of superiority of professional status may make ASW dissent difficult to swallow. Second, they may claim superiority of expertise in this area by confining their definition of relevant knowledge to mental health alone. Third, where two doctors sharing the same perspective agree, they may become more convinced still of the 'incorrectness' of the ASW view.

An inbuilt tension, therefore, exists with an ASW, independent of medical direction, who takes up a social risk orientation. However, our discussion has enabled us to demonstrate further the extent to which the social risk orientation is the 'natural' one for ASWs to take. It is consistent with the 'centre of balance' of their role within the Act; clear analysis through the assessment schedule provides expression for the collective, environmental orientation prevalent in social work; and it further provides expression for, where appropriate, the 'holding' orientation of social work as a whole.

However, the issue is whether this leads to 'creative tension' or conflict between ASWs and doctors. There is a fine line between the two. Creative tension involves the participants using their different perspectives and differing expertise to facilitate and inform the decision-making process. It necessarily involves each giving respect to the other's views. There are good reasons to believe this is a viable hope. ASWs are expected to have two years relevant experience and to have gone through an appropriate training course. The expectation, as a result of this, is the development of some expertise in mental health. A 'spin off' of this expertise is likely to be a greater understanding of the perspectives adopted by doctors and psychiatrists. Furthermore, it would be wrong to over-emphasise the potential for conflict: there may well be quite extensive agreement to start with. Where disagreement occurs, frank discussion may well frequently lead to a shared decision - indeed the legal independence of the decision-makers implies the need for exchange of views before making decisions. Furthermore, research shows, amongst GPs at least, that they perceive ASWs generally to perform their tasks well, which is not so much the case amongst other high profile aspects of social work (Sheppard, 1986; Sheppard, 1987).

Nonetheless, disagreements will occur. Many an ASW will already have experienced, in circumstances where they turned down a section, a doctor saying, threateningly, 'On your head be it'! This is an extremely difficult position to be in, which can only be helped by a clear analysis of the level of the risk and the seriousness of the danger. Furthermore - and despite a general satisfaction amongst GPs with the work of ASWs - the literature is replete with accusations by GPs and psychiatrists of the 'anti-psychiatric' attitude of social workers (Fisher et al, 1984; Bean, 1980). It cannot be emphasised too strongly that the social risk orientation is *not* anti-psychiatric. Instead, it emphasises the need to weigh carefully, clearly and without prior assumptions the risk to an individual *alongside* an assessment of mental disorder. In such a way it becomes possible to make a better assessment of the 'normal' right to liberty against the particular need for treatment.

The ASW Role In Its Wider Context

We have focussed so far exclusively on the role of ASWs in relation to compulsory admissions. This is justified on three grounds: because we have very little information or research-based guidance for ASWs with compulsory admission; because this area is, as has been shown, extremely complex; and because it is important to differentiate the role of the ASW from that of the medical practitioner. It is easy to assume that the ASW, with specialist knowledge of mental health, is in many respects acting simply as a 'poor man's psychiatrist', or to take the erroneous view that the ASW's role is legitimated *solely* by their expertise in examining 'social factors' (however they may be defined). It is only when we understand that social work is concerned with mental health as a social problem, rather than as a health problem *per se,* that this difference begins to emerge.

However, compulsory admission assessments should not be viewed in isolation - discrete events which bear little relationship to the developing social circumstances which precede and succeed these assessments. In our discussion of the assessment schedule, the connection between risks, dangers and patients' social circumstances was explicitly recognised in terms of social support. By working on situations, then, outside (temporally) the formal assessment situation the ASW can have an impact on the assessment itself, either by reducing the likelihood of the need for an assessment or by helping develop in supporters or patients - directly by their own intervention or indirectly by advising others undertaking intervention - abilities which help them manage possible crisis situations better. In the latter case, during an assessment the ASW may be able to mobilise resources which may be personal or material, in the patient or the patient's carers, which avert the need for compulsory admission. In this sense assessments are not discrete occurrences, but part of a wider context. We shall examine this link relating context to assessment in this section.

Compulsory admission assessment is, both in terms of the law and the general consensus of practice, only one aspect - although arguably the most important - of the work of the ASW. The Act itself lays down a number of powers and duties of the ASW, many of which relate to aspects of compulsory admission: for example, the duty to make an application when satisfied it should be made (Section 13(1)), the duty to interview the patient in a suitable manner (Section 13(2)), the duty, when practicable, to inform the nearest relative of a compulsory admission (Section 11(3)) and the power to convey the patient to hospital or to authorise someone else to do so (Section 6(1)). In addition, however, the Act gives the ASW or his Department other powers and duties. Thus, the ASW has the power, among others, to return patients absent without leave (Section 18(1)); powers to enter and inspect premises in which a mentally disordered person lives if they have 'reasonable cause' to believe he is not under proper care (Section 115); the social services authority on request from hospital managers should arrange for a social worker (not necessarily an ASW) to provide a social report for patients where the nearest relative made the application (Section 14); and they have, with the district health authority, the duty to provide aftercare for patients detained under particular sections (Section 117). This is not an exhaustive list, but it indicates that the ASW and the social services authority have responsibilities wider than those simply for compulsory admission. These may be described as related generally to the care of vulnerable mentally disordered people.

However, the ASW is expected to have a wider role than simply reacting to requests for applications for admission to mental hospital, or to ensure the proper legally defined procedures are followed. According to the DHSS Consultative Document produced by the Social Work Services Group in 1981 (Anderson-Ford and Halsey, 1984):

> 'They should have sufficient knowledge and skill to gain the confidence of colleagues in the health services, clients and relatives, and they should fully understand the contribution of members of other disciplines and of the relevant facilities provided by the services for which they work.'

This involves an understanding of patient and family needs, available resources, and the attitudes and contribution of other professionals. The ways in which ASWs are actually used will vary between different authorities, and according to their setting (whether they are in an area team or hospital setting). Broadly, however, a number of potential contributions exist:

1. They can act as adviser or consultant to other colleagues, both in terms of case management, or assessing the mental health state of the client.

2. They can be involved in training and development of other departmental staff.

3. They can be involved in the development of resources for the mentally ill provided by the department, and linking up existing resources where appropriate for mental health needs.

4. They can develop better liaison and collaboration with health professionals, particularly psychiatric.

5. They can improve links with existing voluntary facilities and be involved in the development of new facilities.

The wider role of the ASW may, however, be specifically linked to preventive work in relation to compulsory admissions. In particular the ASW may use their specific expertise to reduce patient vulnerability, concomitantly reducing the need for admission. This can be shown through two examples in which the potential for the use of knowledge-based expertise may provide this link between the wider context and section assessments. The first - using expressed emotion - can be linked to skills with individuals and families, and the second, on depression, emphasises community social work skills.

Psychotic disturbance has been shown consistently to characterise the majority of compulsory admissions. It is well known that schizophrenic patients are very sensitive to their social environment, even when there are no apparent symptoms. The optimal level of arousal may be easily upset if the patient finds him/herself in overstimulating or understimulating social conditions. Thus, over enthusiastic attempts at 'reactivating' unprepared long-stay patients may cause relapse of symptoms, as can occur if a patient is allowed to withdraw too far in an understimulating social environment (Brown et al, 1966). The optimum social environment is structured, with clear-cut realistic roles, and active but neutral supervision to keep up standards of appearance, work and behaviour.

Expressed emotion (EE) refers to the emotions displayed by relatives towards schizophrenic patients, and it has been shown to be significantly related to relapse amongst these patients (Leff and Vaughn, 1984). Three elements have been identified as of particular significance. The level of criticism by the relative of the patient, emotional over-involvement and over-protectiveness, and overt hostility. Those relatives who showed significant levels of these characteristics have been defined as high EE, although critical comments distinguished most high from low EE relatives, and most of the rest manifested emotional over-involvement.

In a number of studies it has been shown that significantly more schizophrenics living with high EE relatives relapse in a given time period than those living with low EE relatives (Brown et al, 1972; Vaughn and Leff, 1976). From this it has been argued that family environment has a significant impact on the course of schizophrenic disorder, with those in low EE families considerably more likely to remain well. Indeed the consistency of these findings in different studies carried out in various countries confirms the pervasive importance of family environment.

An obvious argument about the presence of high EE is that it is understandable given the bizarre behaviour of schizophrenic people: confronted by this behaviour the relative is likely to become tense and irritable, and to feel a considerable level of responsibility for the patient. Indeed, analysis of the content of relatives' criticisms reveals this to be the case in a minority of relatives. However, high EE was related, in the research, primarily to longstanding premorbid interaction between patient and relative. The critical comments made by relatives related, in 70 per cent of cases, less to the specific breakdown than perceived longstanding personality characteristics to do with poor communication or lack of interest shown by the patient. They had always been 'selfish, spoiled, snappy and moody', and the illness merely exacerbated a longstanding, highly unsatisfactory relationship (Leff and Vaughn, 1984).

Leff and Vaughn found that high EE relatives showed particular types of behaviour. They were normally very intrusive, and tried to make contact with the patient when he was quiet and withdrawn, and also tended to disregard requests for privacy, disliking closed doors and patient withdrawal. Second, they tended to be intolerant of the illness, particularly 'sick talk' such as delusional references, and repeatedly engaged in confrontations with the patient, insisting their delusions were just that, leading to tension and arguments. Third, they tended to have high and largely unrealistic expectations of the patient's social functioning and they generally made few allowances for the patient's known deficits, such as underactivity and withdrawal, which could be seen as laziness. This form of behaviour is significant because of schizophrenic patients' vulnerability to 'sensory overload' (Brown et al, 1966). In the face of stressful or socially stimulating circumstances they may well relapse and characteristically withdraw in overstimulating social situations.

Two factors distinguish low EE relatives: they have calm and self-contained responses, sometimes in the face of extremely agitated and bizarre behaviour, and they are extremely flexible in responding to the problems presented by the patient. Although high levels of EE are associated with increased vulnerability to relapse, other factors exert a protective effect, even with high EE. In particular, maintenance drug therapy reduces the likelihood of relapse, as does reduced face-to-face contact between the patient and the high EE relative. Where less than 35 hours' contact occurs each week between patient and high EE relative the patient is considerably less likely to relapse, largely because of the reduced opportunity for hostile interaction to which these patients are vulnerable. It is noteworthy that if the patient and/or relative work, 35 hours represents a large amount of contact: it is necessary for them to spend all the evenings and most of the weekend together to produce this level of contact (Brown et al,1972; Vaughn and Leff, 1976).

Maintenance drug therapy is not, however, sufficient on its own. Another factor inducing relapse is stress-inducing life events, which are presumed to have the same tension-inducing and sensory overloading effects on schizophrenia (Brown and Birley, 1968). When life events occur in a high EE family, their combined effect creates stress too much even for maintenance therapy. As Leff and Vaughn (1984) comment:

> 'Since a threatening event is bound to occur at some point in the patient's life, relapse is only a question of time for those living in high contact with a high EE relative.'

Knowledge of these familial factors is significant in two respects: it provides the basis for prevention of relapse, and it also provides the opportunity for managing situations where relapse occurs that reduces the likelihood of compulsory admission. Two research studies in particular indicate ways of achieving this. The London study of high EE relatives of schizophrenics aimed to achieve *either* a lowering of EE amongst relatives *or* a reduction of face-to-face contact or both (Leff et al, 1982). Three approaches were made: an education programme to increase understanding of patients and their problems; a relatives' group to develop a range of coping behaviour to deal with problems of living with the patient; and family therapy in which problems were worked on by breaking them down into manageable components. Another, even more relevant, study in California involved intervention designed to enhance the effective problem-solving techniques of the family (Falloon et al, 1984). The aim was to use the family as a resource for coping with stressful life events. By developing problem-solving techniques the families would improve their ability to cope with major crises, as well as lesser problems of day-to-day living. This involved six steps, easily recognised by social workers:

1. Identify a specific problem.
2. List alternative solutions.
3. Discuss pros and cons of each solution.
4. Choose the best solution.
5. Plan how to implement the solution.
6. Review efforts.

This approach in an experimental group led to fewer exacerbations of florid symptoms than in the control group and significantly better social functioning.

While these methods reduce the likelihood of relapse, they have significance for ASW compulsory admission assessments in two respects. First, they involve the application of well known social work skills - in education, group and family work. Thus in other contexts social workers attempt to improve coping behaviour, to help improve relatives' understanding of clients' problems, and to improve their problem-solving techniques. In particular the problem-solving techniques resemble both the problem-solving approach of social work, and task-centred work, something implied by Falloon when he referred to 'contingency contracting' as a central part of their work (Perlman, 1957; Reid, 1978; Reid and Epstein, 1972).

Second, they are relevant to the management of compulsory admissions. One of the central elements of assessment discussed in Part Three involved identifying factors reducing the level of risk, in particular focussing on social supports. One element of working with high EE relatives involved helping them cope more flexibly with the patient's bizarre, sometimes difficult behaviour. It should be noted here that many schizophrenic patients, previously hospitalised, retained many of their symptoms, although not sufficiently seriously for hospitalisation. Such symptoms can clearly increase tension in high EE families without the requisite problem-solving abilities. Hence there is a constant potential for relapse. Where successful, these coping techniques would reduce the pressure on relatives themselves, and hence the possible emotional trauma (one criteria for admission identified in the research) when confronted with schizophrenic symptoms. It would in effect increase their coping capacities. Second, development of problem-solving techniques would reduce the impact of life events on the schizophrenic patient, which might otherwise leave them vulnerable, unable to cope, and liable to relapse and admission.

The point here is that at the time of potential crisis it becomes manageable without recourse to admission even when assessment takes place. Having worked on problem-solving techniques the ASW may, with the relative, be able to apply them to the particular situation. This emphasises that work *outside* the particular assessment setting has an impact - the assessment has a wider context. This is because the supports, and hence factors reducing vulnerability (examined in Part Three), may be developed by longer-term work. Furthermore, it involves the use of specialist expertise by the ASW, for we have here called specifically upon research which is the foundation for knowledge-based practice. Hospitalisation, in short, is not simply a matter of mental ill health, but the capacity to cope with it in the community.

A second example relates to depression. A significant element in depression, it is well known, is suicidal feelings, or at least not wishing to live. Depression, therefore, can represent a threat to the patient's safety. However, depression can also have a significant impact on role performance and social functioning. There is, for example, strong evidence linking depression in women to impaired child care performance and relationship and behavioural problems in the children (Weissman and Paykel, 1974). At its extreme a depressed woman may be more violent towards her children, representing a threat to their safety.

Much of the pioneering work of Brown, Harris and their colleagues (1978) is suggestive of ways social workers may work with depression outside the section assessment. It is well established that women are more vulnerable to depression than men (by a ratio of 2:1) (Wiessman and Klerman, 1977). However, Brown and Harris found depression linked also to class: working class women were significantly more likely to become depressed and their depression was more likely to be chronic (i.e. persistent and long lasting) than middle class women. The link between class and depression was made in terms of a number of factors. The first group were provoking agents. These were classified as severe threats - discrete occurrences involving a long-term threat to the subject - and major difficulties, which were ongoing, markedly unpleasant and had lasted at least two years. The events and difficulties covered a wide range of psychological, but not health, factors, such as persistent relationship difficulties, sudden loss (for example, of a job, or a person), financial difficulties, housing difficulties and so on. The working class women experienced more severe events and major difficulties than the middle class women, and some of the social class differences in risk of depression were due to this. These observations will not surprise social workers whose 'bread and butter' involves working with disadvantaged groups, often in appalling conditions, poor housing and general poverty.

However, to explain fully these social class differences a further set of factors was identified. In the overwhelming majority of cases, women only became depressed when experiencing an event or difficulty in the face of an *already existing* vulnerability factor, which interacted with the provoking agent to cause depression. Four were identified: loss of mother before the age of eleven; lack of close confiding relationship with husband or boyfriend; three or more children aged under 14 in the house; and lack of employment. The last of these only became significant if another vulnerability factor was also present. The differences between working class and middle class women, however, were most significantly related to motherhood. Among those with children at home, working class mothers were four times as likely to suffer definite psychiatric disorder as were middle class mothers. Working class women with children aged under six were particularly vulnerable to depression. They were also much more likely to experience a provoking agent.

The interaction then of the events and difficulties they had with the vulnerability presented by their motherhood - particular importance being ascribed to the latter - placed working class women at far greater risk of depression. Furthermore, the numbers were not small: 15 per cent of the Camberwell women suffered a definite affective disorder in the *three months* before being interviewed, while a *further* 18 per cent were considered borderline, possessing definite psychiatric symptoms, but not severe enough to be rated as cases (Brown and Harris, 1978). Indeed, one in four working class mothers suffered definite depression during that period. The working class women suffered significantly more chronic depression, but tended to interpret it socially, perceiving social environment as crucial, and did not seek medical help. Furthermore, in view of the increased number of events experienced by working class mothers, it is significant that the experience of severe events occurring after onset was capable of increasing the depression's severity. Rather than being an isolated marginal problem, depression amongst working class women, largely because of social factors, is of epidemic proportions.

Brown and Harris (1978) pessimistically comment, however, that:

> 'well intentioned intervention in terms of traditional "social work" might not prove very helpful'.

Presumably 'traditional social work' refers to individual casework. It is certainly true that Brown and Harris' research suggests a need for intervention at the level of social policy. However, a broader perception of social work may indeed prove helpful. First, Brown and Harris clearly identify the target group for preventive intervention: working class mothers living in deprived urban areas. This group anyway forms a significant element of social workers' caseloads. Second, work may be undertaken on the basis of two main elements: community social work, through which the women may attempt to gain greater control over their social environment, and the development of problem-solving techniques.

Brown and Harris, drawing on Beck (1967), emphasised the importance of loss and hopelessness in understanding the depression. Loss may not simply be of a person (through, for example, bereavement) but of a role or even an idea. They speculate that the feelings of hopelessness will on occasion become generalised to form the triad of the depressive experience: the feeling that the self is worthless, the future hopeless and the world meaningless. Faced, perhaps, with a loss of great significance, such as the death of a spouse, or problems which appear intractable and increasingly as part of everyday life, the woman may understandably develop an increasing sense of hopelessness and meaninglessness.

Their environment may further engender a sense of helplessness in the face of overwhelming odds. Seligman has, through his theory of 'learned helplessness', developed his view that people denied the opportunity to control their environment in their early years are more likely to react with learned helplessness in adult life (Seligman, 1975; Abramson et al, 1978). This, however, involves a cognitive element - that depression occurs when people perceive themselves in a negative manner as a result of experiencing helplessness. Women, it has been argued, are particularly prone to this, having been socialised to be passive, helpless and dependent, and that their personal worth is dependent considerably on their appeal to men.

These working class mothers in many cases will experience their situation as hopeless, and feel helpless in the face of immense social difficulties. Their desperate life situation confronts them constantly - often living in appalling housing conditions, trying to manage on low incomes, suffering persistent and continual financial problems in an undesirable and sometimes unhygienic environment, often in the most unpleasant of areas. As mothers they have the additional pressure of trying to bring children up adequately, possibly, as Brown and Harris suggest, with less social support than their middle class counterparts, and often without the material resources to provide for quite basic needs.

In view of these dimensions to the women's depression, social work could undertake social intervention designed to give them a greater sense of control over their lives and social environment. The outlines of the approaches suggested here are rather more speculative than those involved with high EE levels, which have the support of research demonstrating effectiveness. However, they do link research evidence with developments in community social work. The Barclay Report identified two types of community social work: that based on locality and that based on a shared concern or problem (National Institute of Social Work, 1982). To a considerable extent, as in Camberwell, location (a poor urban area) and problem (depression in mothers) are linked, helping the social worker focus their intervention more precisely. Community social work, furthermore, is concerned largely with setting up and using social networks and supports.

Social work intervention would be focussed around two main areas: the social environment and child care role. The key to developing a greater sense of control over the social environment is the formation of social networks. This would entail the identification of common problems by the members of these networks in order to begin, as groups, to combat them. These would be identified by the members themselves, with the social worker, and they may involve, for example, poor housing conditions, damp, vandalism or a general neglect and lack of resources. Such an approach has two immediate advantages. First, it involves getting the women's participation, in particular by encouraging them to identify their own problems. Second, it approaches the problems in ways meaningful to the women themselves. As Brown and Harris commented, the women in their study interpreted their depression in social terms, in terms of their disadvantaged environment, and (logically) did not therefore seek medical help. If depression is perceived as a social problem with social causes, then approaching it in that way is likely to elicit more involvement. The second element involves the group(s) themselves identifying those areas which they give the highest priority, and for them to plan and carry out their appropriate response. This involves identifying the various possible solutions, from which the most favoured solution is identified, planning appropriate responses to the solution,identifying the most helpful or appropriate response(s), carrying them out, and evaluating them in terms of whether the goals have been achieved. The participation of the groups themselves in identifying problems, planning action, and carrying out that action is critical if they are to develop a greater sense of control over their lives and environment (as, it must be said, is some degree of success in achieving their goals).

A second area relates to child care. Brown and Harris suggest that, with little support and other problems to manage, the woman perceives herself unable to perform her child care role adequately, and her self-esteem suffers. However, the problems are to a considerable extent environmental rather than simply a reflection on an individual's ability to cope - combining, in particular, extensive social difficulties with the responsibilities for three or more children might be expected to tax most people. In such circumstances the development of child care resources such as creches and play group schemes may be especially valuable for the stressed mother. Further informal supports may be provided where mothers are prepared to share child care responsibilities by, for example, looking after each other's children on occasions where this would be helpful. Where possible, the use and development of social service resources, such as child minding, may be helpful. A critical element of this, apart from its attempt to deal with factors which have a stressful impact on these women, is again its 'self help' - through mutual aid - dimension, which may again serve to emphasise greater control over their circumstances, and which may provide flexible support in the face of problems.

A third element, not dissimilar in this respect to EE, is to enhance the women's problem-solving capacities. Schizophrenic patients are particularly vulnerable to adverse social stimuli, so life events present them with considerable problems. However, life events and difficulties are also significant for depression, although they need to be severe (events) or major (difficulties) in order to have an impact. They would, therefore, be expected to be more difficult to resolve. Some, indeed, may be irresolvable at an individual level - hence the need for community social work.

However, at a group or individual level, problem-solving abilities may be developed for helping the women to manage their problems which do not simply arise because of environmental pressures but because of limitations in their abilities to cope (in admittedly extremely adverse circumstances). Problem-solving, as Perlman (1957) comments, is for helping individuals and families to cope with problems they are currently finding insurmountable, a by-product of which may be learning a way to manage future problems. This involves releasing and giving direction to the client's motivation for change, developing the client's mental, emotional and action capacities, and securing access for the client to helpful resources. It may, for example, be possible through this process to enhance the women's capacity for budget management (although many of them will be in great poverty, this perhaps emphasises the need for good management in view of the absence of any likely added financial help); or to provide help with the management of child care or child behaviour problems. Indeed, working with groups in this way is helpful because of the mutual support they may provide in developing problem-solving techniques and managing problems when they arise.

This approach bears comparison with developments in Haringey described by Ryan (1986). Observing the relationship between social deprivation and female depression, the Social Services Department and Children's Society jointly set up a combination of formal and informal resources. They began by identifying the area of severest deprivation - the Tiverton Estate - and contacted as many tenants as possible through public meetings and informal discussions with special interest groups, such as women with young children or families with teenage children. They found situations creating great stress:

> 'Having the front door kicked in by vandals, but struggling for two years to get it replaced, or being forced, because of severe dampness, to eat and sleep, four in a bed, in one room.'

To deal with this they developed formal resources involving a network of key local agencies, including establishing a local housing office. This encouraged quicker housing repairs, and development of play space and play building in the estate, while the problem of security was met by ansaphone systems.

At the level of familial and social dysfunction the Family Centre was significant. Certain principles guiding the Centre resemble elements already identified, such as participation by the local population, openness to ideas , and respect and encouragement for people's strengths and competencies. The Centre also emphasised an informal social care approach by, for example, using as volunteers local women with their own children to encourage children of depressed mothers to read, and to model a more positive, responsive interactional style between parents and children. In addition, mutual aid networks were developed, such as arranging for babysitters, and providing a place where mothers could meet during the day. The work undertaken in Haringey was described rather than evaluated in terms of its effectiveness in reducing depression and its associated social problems, but its similarity with some of the principles which we have previously described suggests such approaches are realistic.

These approaches may act in a preventive manner. The development of these networks would aim at two effects: to enhance women's sense of control over their environment, and to provide mutual support, both affective and in problem resolution. It would be foolish of course to expect many women in the grip of a severe depression to feel able to take such action. However, such developments do not simply have to involve women who are currently depressed, or even those not currently depressed but vulnerable. Because they tackle issues of wider concern underlying the depression, such action would involve, where successfully organised, others in the community. Where effective in creating a greater sense of control over their environment it would be expected to increase the sense of hope and reduce the incidence of depression. As such, the work would be preventive. Of course, as already suggested, some problems are really so great that they fall into the arena of social policy rather than social work. In certain respects, social work may be seen to be making the 'best of a bad job'.

Both these examples - of schizophrenia and depression - emphasise that psychiatric problems occur in a social context and that ASW assessments cannot be divorced from that context. However, they emphasise also that work outside the assessment context can affect it in two respects: by acting preventively and hence reducing the number of cases where assessments would otherwise have taken place, and by providing appropriate supports which affect the likelihood of admission when assessments actually take place. Furthermore, these examples are knowledge-based, and call upon specialist expertise which the ASW really ought to have.

Social Policy Issues and the Position of the ASW

The activities of ASWs have an even wider context than that of the immediate family or locality; that of social policy relating both to mental health generally and compulsory admission in particular. In approaching this area we have come full circle, because the concept of ASW as gatekeeper is dependent on social policy which grants ASWs their powers and duties through the Mental Health Act. Social policy, then, refers in this context to the legislation and policies which underlie the compulsory admissions, and which governs the circumstances and procedures in which they take place. Thus it is possible to envisage, as with changes from the 1959 Act to the 1983 Act, alterations in the law governing compulsory admissions, or even, in theory, the abolition of compulsory admissions altogether.

The detailed analysis of the interpretation of the 'health or safety of the patient' and 'protection of others' demonstrated the need for greater clarity of analysis by the ASWs undertaking the assessments. However, the wide variations and inconsistencies in interpreting the law are to a considerable degree the result of vagueness in the law itself. It can depend on which ASW and doctor conducts the assessment as to whether or not some patients are compulsorily admitted.

Considerable improvements may be made by the development of methods for clearer analysis. However, the law itself may be made more precise without necessarily infringing greatly on the judgements of the professionals involved in individual situations. The difference between a vague and more precise definition of 'health or safety of the patient' and 'protection of others' is that the latter gives more direction to the worker. In the current situation the 'open texture' of the relevant law is rather *too* open. Furthermore, the lack of any case law, unlike much of the child care law relevant to social work (Hoggett,1987), means that, apart from the guidance of the Mental Health Act Commission, which is not in itself very extensive, little of the 'open texture' has actually been filled in.

The most immediate means for more precise guidance lays with the Secretary of State. Under Section 118 he or she can prepare or revise a code of practice which includes guidance to medical practitioners and approved social workers in relation to admission of patients to hospital, although the Mental Health Act Commission could take action in this respect. It is possible for this guidance to be considerably more precise than that which is currently provided by the law. Any guidance developed could drawn upon the classifications developed in this research to identify circumstances where compulsory admissions should occur. Identifying the conditions to be satisfied for compulsory admission would be far from unique in law relating to social work. Thus, for example, Section 1 of the Children and Young Persons Act 1969 specifies a number of conditions allowing a court to make an order. Of course even these require some interpretation, although the procedure by which a child may be made the subject of a care order differs in at least one significant respect from compulsory admissions: any care order must first go through the due process of law, involving court proceedings, legal representation and court decisions. This model is a 'legal' rather than a 'treatment' model.

In advocating further guidance, this does not necessarily commit us to a 'narrow' interpretation of the law. We do not, for example, have to limit the interpretation of the 'protection of other persons' to injury or death, although this may, in fact, be the decision of the Secretary of State. Indeed, it does not matter - from the point of view of clarity rather than morality - how wide the circumstances are in which a patient may be compulsorily admitted. The point is that the professionals themselves should be clearer about the type of circumstances relevant for admission. Indeed, the patients and nearest relatives may also become clearer about the relevant grounds, providing the opportunity for appeal where it is believed those grounds were not present. It is, furthermore, a matter of openness: the clearer the guidelines, the more honest we are about the way we are treating patients. If, for example, being a nuisance to neighbours falls within the meaning of the Act, by saying so we are not pretending that it is only when the patient is a danger to themselves or others that they are compulsorily admitted. It would add a further dimension to civil rights: for the issue of whether or not disturbing the neighbours provides legitimate grounds for incarcerating any individual, including the mentally disordered, may then be part of the political agenda for social policy. Clarity, in short, aids not just professional conduct, but also civil rights.

The issue, therefore, of whether the ASW should opt for a wide or narrow interpretation of the 'health of the patient' and 'protection of other persons' is bound up with obtaining appropriate guidance, and linked, through the openness and clarity provided by such guidance, to the possibility of civil rights being on the political agenda. This is not to say that it is the job of the ASW to become involved in politics. It is simply that appropriate and open guidance could have a two-fold effect: the improved consistency of ASW practice and the opportunity, if taken up, for a public debate on the legitimate circumstances for compulsory admission.

A second major issue is whether the current provision, involving medical practitioners, approved social workers and nearest relatives having the power to admit the patient compulsorily, is the appropriate one. In this we shall concentrate in particular on the position of the applicant. To a considerable degree this is an issue of professional power, for in 90 per cent of cases it is the ASW who makes the application rather than the nearest relative, leaving both application and medical recommendation entirely in professional hands. Certainly the inconsistency of decision-making does not encourage confidence that patients are always being dealt with fairly, and although partly the result of the legislation itself it also reflects the vagaries of professional practice. Perhaps if ASWs are at times inconsistent the matter should be left in the hands of psychiatrists. Szasz (1963) has drawn attention to the claims made by the American Psychiatric Association that doctors should be able to admit patients unrestricted by other professionals or the courts. Furthermore, as Bean and others have pointed out (Bean, 1980; Wenger and Fletcher, 1969), such a position has a certain logic: if we are committed first and foremost to the treatment of mentally ill patients, then they are either ill or they are not. If they are ill, they should be committed and given treatment as quickly as possible. Such an assertion recognises the claim of psychiatrists to exclusive control of the domain of mental illness.

It is interesting, however, that such a claim leaves the criterion for compulsory admission solely based on mental disorder. There is no place here for issues such as those of the 'health or safety of the patient' or 'protection of others'. Such additional criteria emphasise a position, enshrined in the legislation, that mental disorder alone does not provide sufficient justification for incarcerating an individual (notwithstanding the currently anomalous and inadequately explained position adopted by the Mental Health Act Commission that mental illness be included in the 'health or safety of the patient' criteria). It is therefore clearly the intention of the Act not to regard the domain of compulsory admissions as solely that of the medical profession. The reason for this would appear to be fairly obvious: that the nub of the issue is about whether or not a person should be deprived of their liberty. The question of whether or not a person should be allowed their liberty is not, *per se*, one on which the medical professional can claim any expertise.

This appears to provide a 'space' for others to fill, and it is one taken up by the ASW. Their enhanced position, as already discussed, serves as a means for balancing the tremendous power of medical practitioners. The image of one person, no matter how well intentioned, exercising sole power over whether a person will or will not be compulsorily admitted would certainly appear to many people as somewhat alarming. The presence of the ASW, coming from a different profession, may clearly help to balance this power. Their role, furthermore, appears not simply to be one of assessment but also to encompass a 'watching brief'. Acting, as we have shown, under social auspices is a matter of social concern. ASWs act, as a result, as 'society's representatives'. They are not there because they claim the health domain as their own, although their social science knowledge base may legitimise some claim to expertise. In their role as 'society's representative' they are clearly there to make sure patients are admitted when appropriate, and that they are not admitted when not appropriate. This is consistent with the advice of the Memorandum: that in conducting assessments ASWs must independently consider 'all the circumstances of the case', which include medical opinion. All this serves further to emphasise that the criteria of 'health or safety of the patient' and the 'protection of other persons' provide, to a considerable degree, the key to the ASW's role.

Bean (1980), however, is scathing about social workers in his study of admissions under the 1959 Act:

> 'Social workers', he says, 'have no expertise which qualifies them to do anything except the most simple and basic tasks in the compulsory admissions procedure.

They know less about the patient than the relative and less about psychiatry than the consultant psychiatrist.'

Certainly the training and experience now required of ASWs suggests these criticisms, written before the 1983 Act, are no longer valid. However - and again in the context of the 1983 Act - this misrepresents an important aspect of the ASW role. They are not there simply as experts, although they are expected to have some expertise, but also as 'society's representative' who thus exercises some control over what may otherwise be exclusive medical power. Skills in the assessment of the patient's social circumstances are, of course, important, and if ASWs were incompetent in this respect then they would deserve Bean's criticism. But to rely exclusively on such criticism is to miss the point by perceiving the ASW role as similar to that of the psychiatrist.

Should, however, the whole matter be placed within the formal legal system, a matter for courts and magistrates? This certainly has some merit. It would place the mentally disordered person on a similar footing - procedurally at least - as that of any other person who may be deprived of their liberty. It would, secondly, move the process away from private settings, where justice may be delivered arbitrarily on the whim of individual professionals, into the public arena. Third, it would put them in a setting where issues of justice and liberty are traditionally considered, and where considerable experience about the appropriate circumstances for deprivation of liberty resides.

However, the matter is not that simple. First, it is likely to take more time than currently involved in a compulsory admission in order to go through the process of law. Although the Act discourages unnecessary use of emergency admissions (Section 4) it remains the case that a notable minority of assessments are carried out in crisis situations. If individual magistrates, rather than courts, were approached to speed up this process there is no guarantee that they would provide any greater protection of civil rights than currently exists. Faced with high status experts concerned about dangers presented by and to the patient, the magistrates might find it difficult to resist their requests.

Furthermore, the patients involved are, unless misdiagnosed, suffering from some mental disorder. They may, additionally, frequently be in a sensitive and vulnerable state. As a result they may not be able to appreciate their position or understand what is going on. Even if they do, being made the subject of court proceedings, difficult enough for many people not suffering a mental disorder, is liable to be a traumatic experience. If they are, for example, suffering from paranoid delusions, not uncommon amongst those compulsorily admitted, then the way they view the court may well be influenced by these delusions. In any case, many may run away when threatened with confinement and given time to escape!

We do not have any direct evidence about how such courts would operate in this country, but Fennel's (1977) research on Mental Health Review Tribunals under the 1959 Act may provide some clues. He suggests that:

> 'Where proceedings are organised around familiar legal concepts the legal profession, by virtue of their expertise, exercises a great deal of dominance.'

These proceedings were to consider a patient's fitness for discharge, and involved reports from the psychiatrist as well as the patient who might occasionally be legally represented. The key to the proceedings was the degree of power exerted by the psychiatrist, resulting in the tribunal tending 'to attribute to the legal concepts (of mental disorder, the health or safety of the patients and protection of others) a great deal of elasticity'. The tribunals tended to accept the psychiatrists' judgements, even when contradicted by the patient, except when they were represented and independent corroboration of their version of events was received. It was extremely difficult for the patient to convince the tribunal they were not suffering from mental disorder when contradicted by the psychiatrist. Tribunals were more likely to view the patient in a positive light if they showed 'insight', accepting the psychiatrist's definition of them and the accompanying sick role. Where the issues of the 'health or safety of the patient' or 'protection of others' were concerned there was a tendency to overpredict dangerousness. Hence there was a tendency to predict anti-social conduct in many instances where it was unlikely to occur. These were, of course, proceedings to consider the possible discharge of patients rather than their admission. However, given the similarity of this process to formal legal settings and the apparent dominance in decision-making of the legal profession, this does not inspire confidence that the assessment of psychiatrists would be subject to sufficient critical scrutiny.

The opposite, however, may occur. In the 1960s and 1970s an attempt was made in the United States to insert a legal model within the clinical one. Over the past 20 years there have been numerous test cases resulting from the work of lawyers where patients were released into the community (Anderson-Ford and Halsey, 1984). Considerably influenced by the civil liberties lobby, there developed in American tribunals and courts what has been called 'an obsessive attention to the interpretation of rules' which led to an exhaustive defining and redefining of terminology, which has increasingly resulted in the patient getting off 'on a technicality'. Such a process has not in many cases been in the interests of the patients, particularly in view of the fact that resources have not been adequately provided to ensure proper care and treatment within the community.

All this suggests that courts and legal proceedings are cumbersome and difficult to use where mental disorder and treatment are concerned. The very tension between the need for treatment and the civil liberties of the patients appears to occur in court in ways which favour either one or the other too greatly, and a balance is difficult to achieve. Indeed, the example of the United States suggests that by using courts we can commit an error which is the mirror image of using psychiatrists alone. For while one may tend to emphasise treatment, excluding issues of civil rights, the other, with its emphasis on procedures and technicalities, tends to emphasise civil rights regardless of treatment needs. We are again left with the ASW possessing some mental health expertise, who is prepared and able to examine the 'health or safety of the patient' and 'protection of others' with a great deal of clarity and who is prepared to treat the civil rights of the patient with the utmost seriousness as perhaps the best compromise in this situation.

What, finally, of the nearest relative? Their position, as has already been suggested, is somewhat anomalous in view of the training required by ASWs, and the extensive powers and duties ASWs possess. Although the nearest relative will often have detailed knowledge of the patient, as Bean suggests, this does not mean they are equipped to make an application for compulsory admission. Where the nearest relative lives with, or close to, the patient they will often be the person most disturbed by their behaviour, which may in some cases create legitimate concern for their welfare, but in others simply annoy or frustrate them. Rather than provide a balance to the powers of the medical profession who may want to admit for treatment reasons, the nearest relative may be the person with the greatest stake in getting the patient admitted, whether compulsorily or otherwise. Second, the nearest relative is hardly likely to know the law in any detail, and is unlikely to know, unless guided by the medical practitioner, whether they are acting legally or illegally. Even where guided in this way, they are in no position to know whether this guidance is correct or not: it is difficult, therefore, to say that they are responsible for their decisions in the way that ASWs are. Third, actually making decisions about compulsory admissions is fraught with difficulties. These are difficulties which courts have confronted, and which even they have not been able to resolve by reaching a satisfactory balance between the treatment needs of the patients and their civil rights. It is unlikely that most nearest relatives are going to begin to appreciate these difficulties, let alone take appropriate steps to resolve them. Fourth, the actual assessment process, both of mental disorder and, as we have seen, the 'health or safety of the patient' and 'protection of others' is considerably more complex, and requires greater expertise, than may at first appear. If ASWs, with many years experience, find this problematic we can hardly expect nearest relatives to approach these issues with anything like the clarity and judgement which gives appropriate weight to the patient's civil rights. Finally, the current position, where both ASW *and* nearest relative can be the applicant, far from protecting the patient's civil rights, provides an added opportunity for them to be compulsorily admitted. The author's view is that patients are best served by ASWs being the sole applicant but, as with Section 3 in the current legislation, they can do so only with the agreement of the nearest relative, unless it is impractical or an emergency admission. Should this power be exercised by the nearest relatives, without due regard to the welfare of the patient or the protection of other people, then it should be possible to remove this power by speedy application to the court.

We are left, therefore, with the ASW playing a key role in compulsory admissions. In pursuit of that role, a social risk orientation, and a clear analysis of the relevant criteria are critical if the judgement about mental disorder is to be applied with appropriate consideration of patients' civil rights.

Concluding Comments

This book has had to cover a wide variety of issues in order to get to the heart of the work of the approved social worker. This is, however, no more than a reflection of the great complexity of the role of ASWs, and the situations confronting them when making assessments with a view to possible compulsory admission. This complexity emphatically confirms the need for advanced training which has been taking place following the 1983 Act. It also, however, demonstrates the great importance of the ASW role. All too frequent attacks in the media and the enormous pressures of work have left social workers at times feeling they are involved in a profession under siege, with inevitable effects on their self-esteem as social workers. It is the author's hope that they can take heart from the clear and demonstrable importance of their role as ASWs and be encouraged to achieve the highest possible professional standards.

REFERENCES

Abramson, L., Seligman, M. and Teasdale, J., 1978. Learned helplessness in humans: critique and reformulation, *Journal of Abnormal Psychology,* 87, 49-75.
Akroyd, S. and Hughes, J., 1981. *Data Collection in Context,* London: Longman.
Anderson-Ford, D. and Halsey, M., 1984, *Mental Health Law and Practice for Social Workers,* London: Butterworth.
Barnes, M., Bowl, R. and Fisher, M. (in press). *Sectioned: Social Services and the Mental Health Act 1983,* London: Routledge.
Barnes, M., Bowl, R. and Fisher, M., 1986. The Mental Health Act 1983 and social services, *Research, Policy and Planning,* 4, 1-7.
Bartlett, H., 1970. *The Common Base of Social Work Practice,* Washington DC: National Association of Social Workers.
Bean, P., 1980. *Compulsory Admissions to Mental Hospitals,* London: John Wiley and Sons.
Beck, A., 1967. *Depression: Clinical, Experimental and Theoretical Aspects,* London: Staples Press.
Becker, H., 1963, *Outsiders,* New York: Free Press.
Berger, P. and Luckman, T., 1966. *The Social Construction of Reality,* New York: Doubleday.
Berger, P., 1977. *Pyramids of Sacrifice,* London: Penguin.
Booth, T., Melotte, C., Phillips, D., Pritlove, J. and Lightup, R., 1985. Psychiatric crises in the community: collaboration and the 1983 Mental Health Act. In G. Horobin (ed.), *Responding to Mental Illness,* London: Kogan Page.
Boskoff, A., 1971. Process orientation in sociological theory and research, *Social Forces,* 50, 1-11.
Bowl, R., Barnes, M. and Fisher, M. 1987. A real alternative, *Community Care,* 2 July, 26-28.
Brearley, C., 1984. *Risk and Social Work,* London: Routledge and Kegan Paul.
Brown, G. and Birley, J., 1968. Crisis and life changes and the onset of schizophrenia, *Journal of Health and Social Behaviour,* 9, 203-214.
Brown, G. and Harris, T., 1978. *Social Origins of Depression,* London: Tavistock.
Brown, G. and Rutter, M., 1966. The measurement of family activities and relationships: a methodological study, *Human Relations,* 19, 241-263.

Brown, G., 1987. Social factors and the development and course of depressive disorders in women: a review of a research programme, *British Journal of Social Work,* 17, 615-635.

Brown, G., Bifulco, A. and Harris, R., 1987. Life events, vulnerability and the onset of depression: some refinements, *British Journal of Psychiatry,* 150, 30-42.

Brown, G., Birley, J. and Wing, J., 1972. Influence of family life on the course of schizophrenic disorder: a replication, *British Journal of Psychiatry,* 121, 241-258.

Brown, G., Bone, M., Dalison, B. and Wing, J., 1966. *Schizophrenia and Social Care,* London: Oxford University Press.

Burgess, R., 1984. *In the Field,* London: George Allen and Unwin.

Burrell, G. and Morgan, G., 1979. *Sociological Paradigms and Organisation Analysis,* London: Heinemann.

Butler, A. and Pritchard, C., 1983. *Social Work and Mental Illness,* London: Macmillan.

CCETSW, 1986. *Approved Social Workers. Report of the CCETSW Examinations Board 1984/85,* London: CCETSW.

Christian, L., 1985. *Approved Social Work?* Social Work Monographs, Norwich: UEA Press.

Clare, A., 1980. *Psychiatry in Dissent,* 2nd Edition, London: Tavistock.

Clark, J., 1971. The analysis of crisis management by mental welfare officers, *British Journal of Social Work,* 1, 27-37.

Clinard, M., 1968. *Sociology of Deviant Behaviour,* New York: Holt, Rhinehart and Winston.

Cochrane, R., 1983. *The Social Creation of Mental Illness,* Hong Kong: Longman.

Cohen, A., 1950. The study of social disorganisation and deviant behaviour. In R. Merton, L. Broom and S. Cottrell (eds.), *Sociology Today,* New York: Basic Books.

Corney, R., 1984. *The Effectiveness of Attached Social Workers in the Management of Depressed Female Patients in General Practice,* Cambridge: Cambridge University Press.

Corrigan, P. and Leonard, P., 1978. *Social Work Practice Under Capitalism: A Marxist Approach,* London: Macmillan.

Davies, M., 1981. Social work, the state and the university, *British Journal of Social Work,* 11, 275-288.

Davies, M., 1985. *The Essential Social Worker: A Guide to Positive Practice,* 2nd Edition, Aldershot: Gower.

DHSS, 1983a. *Memorandum on Mental Health Act 1983,* London: HMSO.

DHSS, 1983b. *Mental Health Act 1983: Memorandum on Parts I to VI, VII and X,* London: Department of Health and Social Security.

DHSS, 1985. *The Facilities and Services of Mental Illness and Mental Handicap Hospitals in England, 1982,* London: HMSO.

Edwards, S. and Huxley, P., 1985. A matter of considerable concern, *Community Care,* 28 November.
England, H., 1986. *Social Work as Art,* London: George Allen and Unwin.
Falloon, R., Boyd, J. and McGill, C., 1984. *Family Care of Schizophrenia: A Problem Solving Approach to the Treatment of Mental Illness,* New York: Guildford Press.
Fennel, P., 1977. The Mental Health Review Tribunal: a question of imbalance, *British Journal of Law and Society,* 4, 186-219.
Fisher, M., Barnes, M. and Bowl, R., 1987. Monitoring the Mental Health Act 1983: implications for policy and practice, *Research, Policy and Planning,* 5, 1-7.
Fisher, M., Newton, C. and Sainsbury, E. 1984. *Mental Health Social Work Observed,* London: George Allen and Unwin.
Friedson, E., 1973. *Profession of Medicine,* New York: Dodd and Mead.
Galper, J., 1975. *The Politics of Social Services,* Engelwood Cliffs, NJ: Prentice Hall.
Gibbons, D. and Jones, F., 1975. *The Study of Deviance: Perspectives and Problems,* Englewood Cliffs, NJ: Prentice Hall.
Gilleard, C., 1984. *Living with Dementia,* Hong Kong: Longman.
Goffman, E., 1964. *Behaviour in Public Place,* New York: Free Press.
Goldberg, D. and Huxley, P., 1980. *Mental Illness in the Community: The Pathway to Psychiatric Care,* London: Tavistock.
Goldberg, E. and Warburton, S., 1979. *Ends and Means in Social Work,* London: George Allen and Unwin.
Haines, J., 1975. *Skills and Methods in Social Work,* London: The Trinity Press.
Hardiker, P., 1981. Heart and head - the function and role of knowledge in social work, *Issues in Social Work Education,* 1, 85-111.
Harrison, G., Inechin, B., Smith, J. and Morgan, H., 1984. Psychiatric hospital admissions in Bristol. II: Social and clinical aspects of compulsory admissions, *British Journal of Psychiatry,* 145, 605-611.
Hart, H., 1961. *The Concept of Law,* London: Oxford University Press.
Henderson, A., 1984. Interpreting the evidence on social support, *Social Psychiatry,* 19, 49-52.
Henderson, S., Byrne, D. and Duncan-Jones, P., 1981. *Neurosis in the Social Environment,* London: Academic Press.
Hoggett, B., 1984. *Mental Health Law,* 2nd Edition, London: Sweet and Maxwell.
Hoggett, B., 1987. *Parents and Children: The Law of Parental Responsibility,* 3rd Edition, London: Sweet and Maxwell.
Hoghughi, M., 1980a. *Assessing Problem Children,* London: Sage.
Hoghughi, M., 1980b. Social work in a bind, *Community Care,* 3 April, 17-22.

Mental Health Act Commission, 1987. *Second Biennial Report,* London: HMSO.
Merton, R. and Nisbett, R. (eds.), 1976. *Contemporary Social Problems,* 4th Edition, New York: Harcourt Brace.
Miles, A., 1987. *The Mentally Ill in Contemporary Society,* 2nd Edition, Oxford: Basil Blackwell.
Munro, A. and McCulloch, J., 1969. *Psychiatry for Social Workers,* Oxford: Pergamon.
National Institute of Social Work, 1982. *Social Workers: Their Roles and Tasks,* London: Bedford Square Press.
Parsons, T., 1949. *The Structure of Social Action,* New York: Free Press.
Passamanick, B., Dinitz, S. and Lefton, M., 1959. Psychiatric orientation and its relation of diagnosis and treatment in mental hospital, *American Journal of Psychiatry,* 116, 127-132.
Pavalko, R., 1971. *Sociology of Occupations and Professions,* Illinois: Itasca.
Perlman, H., 1957. *Social Casework: A Problem Solving Process,* Chicago: University of Chicago Press.
Phillips, D., 1983, Mayer and Timms revisited. In M. Fisher (ed.), *Speaking of Clients,* Sheffield: Joint Unit for Social Services Research, University of Sheffield.
Platt, S., 1981. Social adjustment as a criterion of treatment success: just what are we measuring? *Psychiatry,* 44, 95-112.
Rack, P., 1982. *Race, Culture and Mental Disorder,* London: Tavistock.
Raynes, N., 1980. A preliminary study of search procedures and patient management techniques in general practice, *Journal of the Royal College of General Practitioners,* 30, 166-172.
Rees, S., 1978. *Social Work Face to Face,* London: Edward Arnold.
Reid, W. and Epstein, L., 1972. *Task Centred Casework,* New York: Columbia University Press.
Reid, W., 1978. *The Task Centred System,* New York: Columbia University Press.
Rowe, W., 1977. *An Anatomy of Risk,* London: John Wiley.
Rutter, M. and Brown, G., 1966. The reliability of family life and relationships in families containing a psychiatric patient, *Social Psychiatry,* 1, 38-53.
Ryan, P., 1986. The contribution of formal and informal systems to the alleviation of depression in young mothers, *British Journal of Social Work,* Supplement, 71-83.
Scheff, T., 1984. *Being Mentally Ill: A Sociological Theory,* 2nd edition, Chicago: Aldine.
Seligman, M., 1975. *Helplessness,* San Francisco: Freeman.
Sheldon, B., 1978. Theory and practice in social work: a re-examination of a tenuous relationship, *British Journal of Social Work,* 8, 1-21.

Sheldon, B., 1983. The use of single case experimental designs in the evaluation of social work, *British Journal of Social Work*, 13, 477-499.
Shepherd, M., Harwin, B., Depla, C. and Cairns, V., 1979. Social work and the primary care of mental disorder, *Psychological Medicine*, 9, 661-669.
Sheppard, M., 1982. *Perceptions of Child Abuse: A Critique of Individualism*, Social Work Monographs, Norwich: UEA Press.
Sheppard, M., 1984. Notes on the use of social explanation to social work, *Issues in Social Work Education*, 4, 1, 27-42.
Sheppard, M., 1986. Primary health care workers' views about social work, *British Journal of Social Work*, 16, 459-468.
Sheppard, M., 1987. Dominant images of social work: a British comparison of general practitioners with and without attachment schemes, *International Social Work*, 30, 77-91.
Sheppard, M., 1988. The diagnosis of black schizophrenics in Britain, *The Guardian*, 7 November.
Sibeon, R., 1982. Theory-practice symbolisation: a critical review of the Hardiker/Davies debate, *Issues in Social Work Education*, 2, 119-147.
Sims, A. and Symonds, R., 1975. Psychiatric referrals from the police, *British Journal of Psychiatry*, 127, 171-178.
Smuckler, G., Bird, A. and Button, E., 1981. Compulsory admissions in a London borough. 1. Social and clinical features and follow up, *Psychological Medicine*, 11, 617-636.
Smuckler, G.,1981. Compulsory admissions to a London borough. II. Circumstances surrounding admission - service implications, *Psychological Medicine*, 11, 025-039.
Stevenson, O. and Parsloe, P., 1978. *Social Service Teams: The Practitioner's View*, London: HMSO.
Strasser, H., 1976. *The Normative Structure of Sociology*, London: Routledge and Kegan Paul.
Szasz, T., 1961. *The Myth of Mental Illness*, New York: Harper.
Szasz, T., 1963. *Law, Liberty and Psychiatry*, London: Macmillan.
Vaughn, C. and Leff, J., 1976. The influence of family and social factors on the course of psychiatric illness: a comparison of schizophrenic and depressed patients, *British Journal of Psychiatry*, 29, 125-137.
Veiel, H., 1985. Dimensions of social support: a conceptual framework for research, *Social Psychiatry*, 20, 156-162.
Weber, M., 1946, *Essays in Sociology*, London: Oxford University Press.
Weissman, M. and Klerman, G., 1977. Sex differences and the epidemiology of depression, *Archives of General Psychiatry*, 34, 98-111.

Weissman, M. and Paykel, E., 1974. *The Depressed Woman: A Study of Social Relationships,* Chicago: University of Chicago Press.

Wenger, D. and Fletcher, C., 1969. The effect of legal counsel and admissions to a state mental hospital: a confrontation of professions, *Journal of Health and Social Behaviour,* 10, 66-72.

White-Franklin, A. (ed.), 1977. *The Challenge of Child Abuse,* London: Academic Press.

Wilding, P., 1982. *Professional Power and Social Welfare,* London: Routledge and Kegan Paul.

Wing, J., Birley, J., Cooper, J., Graham, R. and Isaacs, A., 1967. Reliability of a procedure for measuring and classifying 'present psychiatric state', *British Journal of Psychiatry,* 113, 449-515.

Woof, K., 1987. *A Comparison of the Work of Community Psychiatric Nurses and Mental Health Social Workers in Salford,* Ph.D. Thesis, University of Manchester.

World Health Organisation, 1977. *Manual of the International Statistical Classification of Diseases, Injuries and Causes of Death,* (9th Revision), Volume 1, London: HMSO.